COPYCAT RECIPES
&
COPYCAT RESTAURANT FAVORITES

{2 Books in 1}

A Complete Compilation of the Most Famous Healthy and Low-Carb Recipes That you can Cook Comfortably at Your Own Home with an Instant Success!

Melissa Pot

~ TABLE OF CONTENTS ~

BOOK 1 :

"COPYCAT RECIPES"

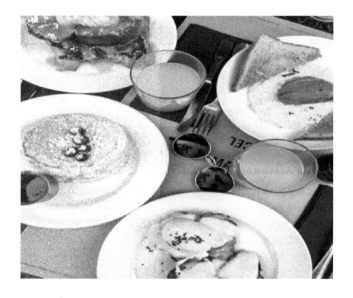

BOOK 2 :

"COPYCAT RESTAURANT FAVORITES"

9

MELISSA POT

COPYCAT

RECIPES

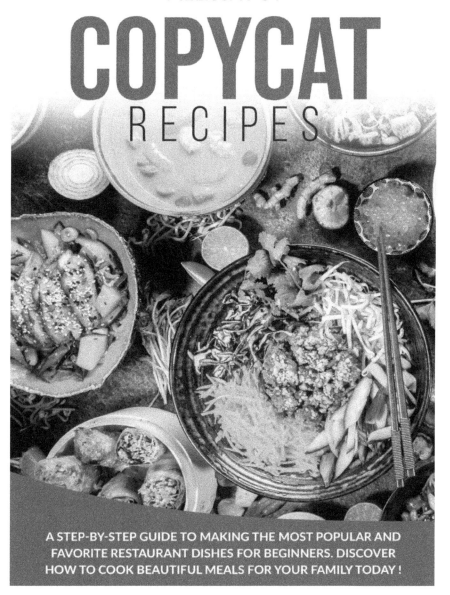

COPYCAT RECIPES

A Step-by-Step Guide to Making the Most Popular and Favorite Restaurant Dishes for Beginners. Discover how to Cook Beautiful Meals for Your Family Today !

Melissa Pot

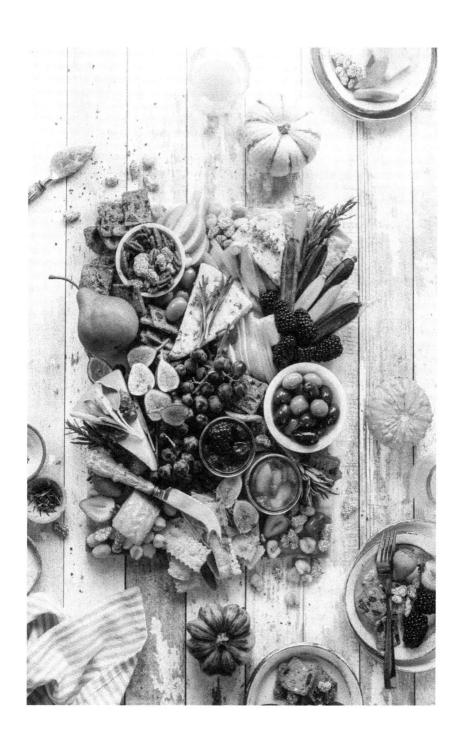

Introduction

American families adore going out to eat at their favorite restaurants; however, surveys have shown that people are spending less money than ever at restaurants due to budget restrictions and a declining economy. If you are one of those people, why not surprise your family and friends with their favorite restaurant dish by making it at home in your own kitchen?

In reading this, you will realize that you can actually cook at home the recipes that you love the most for a fraction of the cost of dining out. You will find step-by-step instructions for all those amazing dishes that draw people into restaurants, and you will be sure that the food was cooked under hygienic conditions since you will be making it yourself.

You don't have to be a master chef to prepare these meals. All these recipes use basic ingredients that can be found in any grocery store.

Here, you will find tips on how to create the restaurant feeling at home. You'll get a list of basic cookware and appliances you need to have in your kitchen as well as how to stock your pantry to prepare some amazing dishes. There will be a primer on how to choose the best and freshest ingredients. You will also learn the basic cooking terms and techniques used in here.

The Cost of Eating Out

When you pay for a meal at a restaurant, usually you're paying three times more than the actual cost of the ingredients it took to make the food. That's around $14 in a restaurant which would have only cost $4.25 if you had made it yourself. There are four ways restaurant owners' price their menu items. "Cost of raw ingredients" divided by "desired food cost percentage (which is about 25-30%)" equals "the price." This is how the $14 restaurant meal cost was calculated earlier.

The second method is to base the price on competing restaurants. Restaurant owners will either adopt the same price of their competitors, lower the price of their meals for those trying to find a better deal, or raise their prices to appear of higher quality compared to their competition.

The third method of menu pricing is to base prices on supply and demand. For example, the food is usually priced higher at places like sports stadiums and airports simply because they know you will be hungry and thirsty and there aren't a lot of other options. Restaurants that have unique themes to their interior or food can also mark their prices higher since the customers aren't just paying for the food, they're also paying for the overall dining experience.

Finally, the fourth and last pricing method is by evaluating your menu items' profitability. If restaurant owners know that one particular meal is selling well, they will raise the other prices by just a small, infinitesimal amount so that it will increase profitability to balance with the best-sellers. Regardless of the pricing method, when you're eating at a restaurant, you're not just paying for the food but for the restaurants overhead as well.

Copycat restaurant recipes are now widely known because of the ever-high cost of eating out. These copycat restaurant recipes are the hidden recipes from all your favorite restaurants in America so you can prepare them in the comfort of your home.

The benefit of using copycat restaurant recipes is that not only can you save money; you can also customize the recipes. For example, if you want to reduce the salt or butter in one of the plates, you can. Now you've saved money, and at the same time provided a nutritious meal for your family.

You have little control over the ingredients in the meal when you eat out. You can't, of course, adjust the dish that you order because sauces, etc. are made in advance.

All of us know that it is expensive to take our family out for dinner, and without a doubt, this would easily cost you around a hundred dollars on an average. With copycat restaurant recipes the same one hundred dollars can easily produce 4 or more meals.

Now, imagine that you also have all the needed ingredients at home for a second to cook the same food with copycat restaurant recipes. So, when you're making a copycat restaurant recipe you can "wow" your family and guests.

You're going to have them thinking you've picked up dinner from a favorite restaurant just by using these recipes and saving costs compared to dining out.

Trying to guess what the ingredients are to your favorite restaurant meal is eliminated when you use copycat recipes. You simply follow the recipe, and slowly recreate your favorite meal.

Having regular meals inspired by your favorite restaurants as a family allows for a healthier, more tight-knit family. Research have shown that in school, families who dine together at home are more united, happier and the kids perform better.

To sum up, the huge savings you'll gain from cooking at home could be used for more productive things like a family holiday or college tuition for your kids.

Going out for a meal at your favorite restaurant is always fun to most. But what if you had access to the top-secret restaurant recipes that so heavily guard those popular restaurants? Would you go home cooking these yourself whenever you wish?

It is not really that difficult to learn how to cooktop secret restaurant recipes. Some think you need a degree in culinary arts or cooking education so you can cook those secret recipes. I hate telling you this, but anyone can collect the ingredients themselves and cook a fancy meal that tastes like the real thing.

But do top secret restaurant recipes really taste the way the chef served them? Perhaps. You can easily cook your favorite recipes with a little practice and patience.

The advantage of making your own top-secret recipes is that you can add to your recipes your own flavors and spices. You'd just want to cook the basic formula and start adding what you think would make the flavor of the recipe better after a while. You may start to figure out that some recipes might need a little more herbs or peppers to make the dish better than the original!

Cooking top secret recipes from restaurants will also make your friends and family wonder where you've learned to cook so well. Imagine cooking a whole meal that looks like it was the restaurant's take-out food. I bet some friends of yours won't even believe you've cooked it!

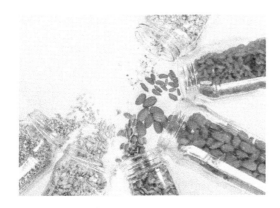

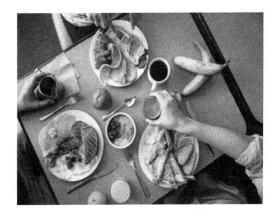

Famous Breakfast Recipes

Spinach and Cheese Egg Soufflé from Panera

Preparation Time: 15

Cooking Time: 25

Servings: 4

Ingredients:

1 tube butter flake crescent rolls

6 eggs, divided

2 tablespoons milk

2 tablespoons heavy cream

¼ cup cheddar cheese, grated

¼ cup jack cheese, grated

1 tablespoon Parmesan cheese

3 tablespoons fresh spinach, mince

4 slices of bacon, cooked and crumbled

Cooking spray

¼ teaspoon salt

¼ cup Asiago cheese, grated, divided

Directions:

Preheat oven to 375°F.

Add 5 eggs, milk, heavy cream, cheddar cheese, jack cheese, parmesan cheese, spinach, bacon, and salt to a nonreactive bowl. Mix well until combined then heat in microwave for about 30 seconds. Stir, then microwave for another 20 seconds. Repeat about 5 times or until egg mixture is a bit thicker but still runny and uncooked.

Roll out crescent roll dough. Make 4 rectangles by pressing together the triangles. Then, using a roll pin, stretch them out until they are 6in x 6in square.

Coat ramekin with cooking spray and place flattened roll inside, making sure the edges are outside the ramekin. Add ⅓ cup egg mixture and then about ⅛ cup Asiago cheese. Wrap edges of the roll-on top. Repeat for remaining rolls.

Whisk remaining egg with salt lightly in a bowl then, with a pastry brush, brush on top of each crescent roll dough.

Place ramekins in the oven and bake for 20 minutes or until brown.

Serve.

Nutrition:

Calories: 303, Fat: 25 g, Saturated Fat: 11 g, Carbs: 4 g, Sugar: 1 g, Fibers: 0 g, Protein: 20 g, Sodium: 749 mg

Sonic's SuperSONIC™ Copycat Burrito

Preparation Time: 10 minutes

Cooking Time: 25 minutes

Servings: 8

Ingredients:

50 tater tots, frozen

1-pound breakfast sausage patties - 8 large eggs, beaten

2 tablespoons half and half - Salt and pepper, to taste

1 tablespoon butter - 8 6-inch flour tortillas

1½ cups cheddar cheese, grated - 1 medium onion, diced

½ cup pickled jalapeño peppers, sliced - 3 roma tomatoes, sliced

Salsa

Directions: Cook tater tots per instructions on the package but cook them so they are a bit crispy. Set aside. In a pan, cook sausage patties. Break apart into large clumps until brown.

Add eggs, half and half, salt, and pepper in a bowl. Whisk until well mixed.

Heat butter in a pan over medium heat. Pour egg mixture and stir every now and then until scrambled Remove from heat.

Microwave tortillas until warm but still soft. Then, in a vertical line in the center, add cheddar cheese, eggs, cooked sausage, tater tots, onions, jalapeños, and tomato. Fold the ingredients using the outer flaps of the tortilla. Repeat with remaining ingredients and tortillas.

Serve warm with salsa.

Nutrition: Calories: 636, Fat: 40 g, Saturated Fat: 16 g, Carbs: 39 g, Sugar: 4 g, Fibers: 3 g, Protein: 28 g, Sodium: 1381 mg

Cracker Barrel's Biscuits

Preparation Time: 15 minutes

Cooking Time: 8 minutes

Servings: 8

Ingredients:

2 cups self-rising flour

⅓ cup shortening

⅔ cup buttermilk

Melted butter, to brush

Directions:

Preheat oven to 450 °F.

In a bowl, mix flour and shortening until mixture is loose and crumbly.

Pour in buttermilk. Mix well.

Sprinkle flour onto a smooth surface and flatten dough on top. Cut dough into desired shapes using biscuit cutters.

Arrange onto a baking sheet. Place in oven and cook for 8 minutes. Apply melted butter on top using a brush.

Serve.

Nutrition: Calories: 194, Fat: 9 g, Carbs: 24 g, Protein: 4 g, Sodium: 418 mg

The Spinach and Artichoke Dip from Applebee's

Preparation Time: 5 minutes

Cooking Time: 30 minutes

Servings: 10

Ingredients:

1 10-ounce bag spinach, diced

2 14-ounce cans artichoke hearts, diced

1 cup Parmesan-Romano cheese mix, grated

2 cups mozzarella cheese, grated

16 ounces garlic alfredo sauce

8 ounces cream cheese, softened

Directions:

Combine all ingredients in a bowl. Mix well.

Transfer into a slow cooker. Set on high and cook for 30 minutes.

Serve while hot.

Nutrition: Calories: 228, Fat. 15 g, Carbs: 12 g, Protein: 13 g, Sodium: 418 mg

Copycat Mozzarella Sticks from TGI Fridays

Preparation Time: 10 minutes

Cooking Time: 5 minutes

Servings: 16

Ingredients:

⅔ cup all-purpose flour

2 large eggs

¼ cup milk

1 cup Japanese breadcrumbs

½ cup Parmesan cheese, shredded

1 tablespoon dried parsley

½ teaspoon garlic salt

½ teaspoon seasoning salt

8 pieces mozzarella string cheese

1-quart vegetable oil

Marinara sauce

Directions:

Add flour to a bowl. Then, in a separate bowl, mix eggs and milk. Add breadcrumbs, Parmesan, parsley, garlic salt, and seasoning salt in a third bowl and mix well.

Line baking sheet with wax paper. Set aside.

Cut mozzarella pieces in half vertically so that you will end up with 16 mozzarella sticks. Then, for each piece, dredge first in flour, followed by egg wash, and third in breadcrumb mixture. Dredge again in egg wash and breadcrumbs for a thicker coat. Place pieces on prepared baking sheet and place in freezer for at least 1 hour or overnight.

To prepare mozzarella sticks preheat deep fryer to 350°F.

About 4 sticks at a time, deep fry for about 30 seconds or until golden brown. Using a slotted spoon, transfer to a rack or plate lined with paper towels to drain.

Serve warm with marinara sauce.

Nutrition: Calories: 118, Fat: 7 g, Saturated Fat: 4 g, Carbs: 8 g, Sugar: 1g, Fiber: 0g, Protein: 7 g, Sodium: 340 mg

The French Toasts from Denny's

Preparation Time: 10 minutes

Cooking Time: 12 minutes

Servings: 6

Ingredients:

Batter:

4 eggs

⅔ cup whole milk

⅓ cup flour

⅓ cup sugar

½ teaspoon vanilla extract

¼ teaspoon salt

⅛ teaspoon cinnamon

Other ingredients

6 slices bread loaf, sliced thick

3 tablespoons butter

Powdered sugar for dusting

Syrup as desired

Directions:

Mix in the ingredients for batter in a bowl.

Soak bread slices in batter one at a time for at least 30 seconds on both sides. Allow excess batter to drip off. Melt 1 tablespoon of butter in a pan, cook battered bread over medium heat for 2 minutes or until each side is golden brown. Move slice to a plate.

Repeat with the remaining slices of bread, adding more butter to the pan if needed.

Dust with powdered sugar, if desired, and with syrup poured on top.

Nutrition: Calories: 264, Fat: 11 g, Carbs: 33 g, Protein: 8 g, Sodium: 360 mg

IHOP's Healthy "Harvest Grain 'N Nut" Pancakes

Preparation Time: 5 minutes

Cooking Time: 5 minutes

Servings: 4

Ingredients:

1 teaspoon olive oil - ¾ cup oats, powdered

¾ cup whole wheat flour - 2 teaspoons baking soda

1 teaspoon baking powder - ½ teaspoon salt

1½ cup buttermilk - ¼ cup vegetable oil - 1 egg - ¼ cup sugar

3 tablespoons almonds, finely sliced

3 tablespoons walnuts, sliced

Syrup for serving

Directions: Heat oil in a pan over medium heat.

As pan preheats, pulverize oats in a blender until powdered. Then, add to a large bowl with flour, baking soda, baking powder and salt. Mix well.

Add buttermilk, oil, egg, and sugar in a separate bowl. Mix with an electric mixer until creamy.

Mix in wet ingredients with dry ingredients, then add nuts. Mix everything together with electric mixer.

Scoop ⅓ cup of batter and cook in the hot pan for at least 2 minutes or until both sides turn golden brown. Transfer onto a plate, then repeat for the remaining batter. Serve with syrup.

Nutrition: Calories: 433, Fat: 24 g, Carbs: 46 g, Protein: 12 g, Sodium: 1128 mg

McDonald's Sausage Egg McMuffin

Preparation Time: 10 minutes

Cooking Time: 15 minutes

Servings: 4

Ingredients:

4 English muffins, cut in half horizontally

4 slices American processed cheese

½ tablespoon oil

1-pound ground pork, minced

½ teaspoon dried sage, ground

½ teaspoon dried thyme

1 teaspoon onion powder

¾ teaspoon black pepper

¾ teaspoon salt

½ teaspoon white sugar

4 large ⅓-inch onion ring slices

4 large eggs

2 tablespoons water

Directions:

Preheat oven to 300°F.

Cover one half of muffin with cheese, leaving one half uncovered. Transfer both halves to a baking tray. Place in oven.

For the sausage patties, use your hands to mix pork, sage, thyme, onion powder, pepper, salt, and sugar in a bowl. Form into 4 patties. Make sure they are slightly larger than the muffins.

Heat oil in a pan. Cook patties on both sides for at least 2 minutes each or until all sides turn brown. Remove tray of muffins from oven. Place cooked sausage patties on top of the cheese on muffins. Return tray to the oven.

In the same pan, position onion rings flat into a single layer. Crack one egg inside each of the onion rings to make them round. Add water carefully into the sides of the pan and cover. Cook for 2 minutes.

Remove tray of muffins from the oven. Add eggs on top of patties, then top with the other muffin half.

Serve warm.

Nutrition: Calories: 453, Fat: 15 g, Carbs: 67 g, Protein: 15 g, Sodium: 1008 mg

Starbucks' Spinach and Feta Breakfast Wraps

Preparation Time: 5 minutes

Cooking Time: 20 minutes

Servings: 6

Ingredients:

10 ounces spinach leaves

1 14½-ounce can dice tomatoes, drained

3 tablespoons cream cheese - 10 egg whites - ½ teaspoon oregano

½ teaspoon garlic salt - ⅛ teaspoon pepper

6 whole wheat tortillas - 4 tablespoons feta cheese, crumbled

Cooking Spray

Directions:

Apply light coating of cooking spray to a pan. Cook spinach leaves on medium-high heat for 5 minutes or until leaves wilt, then stir in tomatoes and cream cheese. Cook for an additional 5 minutes or until cheese is melted completely. Remove from pan and place into glass bowl and cover. Set aside.

In the same pan, add egg whites, oregano, salt, and pepper. Stir well and cook at least 5 minutes or until eggs are scrambled. Remove from heat.

Microwave tortillas for 30 seconds or until warm. Place egg whites, spinach and tomato mixture, and feta in the middle of the tortillas. Fold sides inwards, like a burrito. Serve.

Nutrition: Calories: 157, Fat: 3 g, Carbs: 19 g, Protein: 14 g, Sodium: 305 mg

Jimmy Dean's Homemade Pork Sage Sausage

Preparation Time: 5 minutes

Cooking Time: 20 minutes

Servings: 4

Ingredients:

1-pound ground pork

1 teaspoon salt

½ teaspoon dried parsley

¼ teaspoon rubbed sage

¼ teaspoon black pepper, ground

¼ teaspoon dried thyme

¼ teaspoon coriander

¼ teaspoon seasoned salt

Directions:

Mix all ingredients in a bowl.

Shape into patties. Then, cook in a pan on medium heat until meat is brown on both sides and cooked through.

Serve.

Nutrition: Calories: 313, Fat: 24 g, Carbs: 4 g, Protein: 19 g , Sodium: 646 mg

Baked Oatmeal for a Crowd with Berries and Seeds

Preparation Time: 20 minutes

Cooking Time: 50 minutes

Servings: 8

Ingredients:

4 tablespoons unsalted butter, melted, plus more for pan

6 medjool dates, pitted and chopped (1/2 cup)

4 cups old fashioned rolled oats - 1 teaspoon baking powder

1/2 teaspoon kosher salt - 1/2 teaspoon ground cinnamon

4 cups whole milk - 1/4 cup pure maple syrup, plus more

for serving

2 large eggs - 2 teaspoons pure vanilla extract

1 cup fresh or frozen mixed berries - 1/4 cup toasted pepitas

2 tablespoons hemp seed hearts

Directions:

Step 1: Heat oven to 350°F. Butter a 3-quart baking dish. Sprinkle dates evenly along bottom. In a large bowl, whisk together oats, baking powder, salt, and cinnamon. In another bowl, combine milk, maple syrup, melted butter, eggs, and vanilla extract. Add to bowl with oats and stir to combine. Transfer to prepared dish.

Step2: Sprinkle top with berries and bake until just set, about 35 minutes. Sprinkle pepitas and hemp hearts over oatmeal. Let cool 20 minutes. Serve warm or cold with extra maple syrup, if desired. Baked oatmeal can be stored covered in the refrigerator up to 5 days.

Nutrition: Calories: 312, Fat: 26g, Carbs: 4g, Protein: 18 g, Sodium: 356g

DIY California A.M. Crunchwrap

Preparation Time: 10 minutes

Cooking Time: 20 minutes

Servings: 4

Ingredients:

4 frozen hash brown patties

5 large eggs - 1 tablespoon milk

Salt and pepper, to taste

4 large tortillas - 1 cup cheddar cheese, shredded

4 strips of thick cut bacon, cooked and crumbled

2 ripe California avocados, peeled and pitted

4 tablespoons pico de gallo

Directions:

Cook hash brown patties until crisp, based on package instructions.

Add eggs, milk, salt, and pepper in a bowl. Mix well until combined. Then, pour onto a skillet and cook until scrambled. Set aside.

Heat two different-sized (one smaller than other) heavy bottomed pans over medium heat. Once heated, place tortillas into the bigger pan and, in even amounts, add cheese, a hash brown patty, eggs, bacon, avocado, and pico de gallo in the center of the tortilla in that order.

Using a wheel pattern, fold tortilla around the filling with the edge facing up. Place heated smaller pan (such as a cast iron skillet) on top for about 20 seconds or until browned. Serve immediately.

Nutrition: Calories: 933, Fat: 51 g, Saturated Fat: 15 g, Carbs: 91 g, Sugar: 1 g, Fibers: 11 g, Protein: 32 g, Sodium: 1343 mg

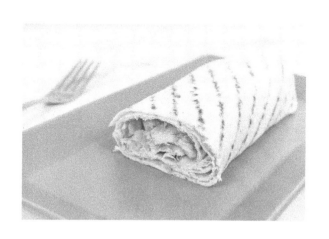

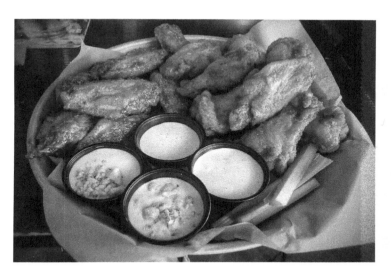

Appetizers I

Pei Wei's Crab Wonton

Preparation Time: 10 minutes

Cooking Time: 5 minutes

Servings: 6

Ingredients:

1 (7-ounce) can white crab meat

½ pound cream cheese, softened

2-3 green onions, sliced

½ tablespoon garlic powder

Splash of soy sauce

Wonton wrappers

Cooking oil

Directions:

Combine the crab, cream cheese, green onions, garlic powder and soy sauce in a bowl. Stir until the mixture reaches a paste-like consistency.

Spoon a bit of the mixture into each wonton wrapper and fold. Seal around the edges with a moistened finger.

Nutrition: Calories: 244, Fat: 15 g, Carbs: 34 g, Protein: 87 g, Sodium: 344 g

Pei Wei's Vietnamese Chicken Salad Spring Roll

Preparation Time: 10 minutes

Cooking Time: 1 minutes

Servings: 4-6

Ingredients:

Salad

Rice Wrappers

Green leaf lettuce like Boston Bibb lettuce

Napa cabbage, shredded

Green onions, chopped

Mint, chopped

Carrots, cut into 1-inch matchsticks

Peanuts

Chicken, diced and cooked, about 6 chicken tenders drizzled with soy sauce, honey, garlic powder, and red pepper flakes

Lime dressing

2 tablespoons lime juice, about 1 lime

1½ teaspoons water

1 tablespoon sugar

1 teaspoon salt

Dash of pepper

3 tablespoons oil

Add everything but the oil to a small container or bowl and shake or stir until the sugar and salt are dissolved. Next, add the oil and shake well.

Peanut dipping sauce

2 tablespoons soy sauce

1 tablespoon rice wine vinegar

2 tablespoons brown sugar

¼ cup peanut butter

1 teaspoon chipotle Tabasco

1 teaspoon honey

1 teaspoon sweet chili sauce

1 teaspoon lime vinaigrette

Add all the ingredients to a small bowl and mix to combine thoroughly.

Directions:

In a large bowl, mix together all of the salad ingredients except for the rice wrappers and lettuce.

Place the rice wrappers in warm water for about 1 minute to soften.

Transfer the wrappers to a plate and top each with 2 pieces of lettuce.

Top the lettuce with the salad mixture and drizzle with the lime dressing. Fold the wrapper by tucking in the ends and then rolling.

Serve with lime dressing and peanut dipping sauce.

Nutrition: Calories: 178, Fat: 4.4 g, Carbs: 7 g, Protein: 68 g, Sodium: 357 g

Takeout Dry Garlic Ribs

Preparation Time: 15 minutes

Cooking Time: 2 hours and 15 minutes

Servings: 4-6

Ingredients:

6 pounds pork ribs, silver skin removed and cut into individual ribs

1½ cups broth - 1½ cups brown sugar - ¼ cup soy sauce

12 cloves garlic, minced - ¼ cup yellow mustard

1 large onion, finely chopped - ¼ teaspoon salt

½ teaspoon black pepper

Directions: Preheat oven to 200°F.

Season ribs with salt and pepper and place on a baking tray. Cover with aluminum foil and bake for 1 hour.

In a mixing bowl, stir together the broth, brown sugar, soy sauce, garlic, mustard and onion. Continue stirring until the sugar is completely dissolved.

After an hour, remove the foil from the ribs and turn the heat up to 350°F.

Carefully pour the sauce over the ribs. Re-cover with the foil and return to the oven for 1 hour.

Remove the foil and bake for 15 more minutes on each side.

Nutrition: Calories: 233, Fat: 3.6 g, Carbs: 6.4 g, Protein:65 g, Sodium: 434 g

Abuelo Jalapeno Poppers

Preparation Time: 10 minutes

Cooking Time: 1 hour and 10 minutes

Servings: 8

Ingredients:

30 jalapeno peppers; sliced into half lengthwise

1 cup milk

2 packages soften cream cheese, at room temperature (8-ounces each)

1/8 teaspoon paprika

12 ounces Cheddar cheese, shredded

1/8 teaspoon chili powder

1 cup flour

1/8 teaspoon garlic powder

1 cup seasoned breadcrumbs

1/4 teaspoon ground black pepper

1 quart of oil for frying

1/4 teaspoon salt

Directions:

Scrape out seeds and the pith inside of the jalapeno peppers using a spoon. Combine cheddar cheese together with cream cheese in a medium-sized bowl; give them a good stir until blended well. Fill each pepper half with the prepared cream cheese blend using a spoon.

Add flour into a small-sized shallow bowl. Add paprika, pepper, garlic powder, chili powder and salt. Blend into the flour until it is mixed. Pour milk into a separate medium-sized shallow bowl. Dip stuffed jalapeno into flour. Place the floured pepper on a large-sized baking sheet with a rack. Let dry for 10 minutes.

Pour the dried breadcrumbs into a separate bowl. Dip the floured jalapeno pepper into the milk & then into the bowl with the breadcrumbs. Place the pepper on the rack again. Preheat the oil to 350 F in advance. Dip pepper into the milk & then into the breadcrumbs. Repeat these steps until you have utilized the entire dipping peppers.

Work in batches and fry peppers for a minute or two, until turn golden brown. Remove from oil & place them on a baking rack to drain.

Nutrition: Calories: 257, Fat: 14. 3 g, Carbs: 18.9 g, Protein: 21.5, Sodium: 531 mg

Applebee's Baja Potato Boats

Preparation Time:10 minutes

Cooking Time: 30 minutes

Servings: 4

Ingredients:

For Pico de Gallo: 1 ½ teaspoon fresh cilantro, minced

1 tablespoon canned jalapeño slices (nacho slices), diced

3 tablespoons Spanish onion, chopped

1 chopped tomato (approximately ½ cup)

A dash each of freshly-ground black pepper & salt

For the Potato Boats:

2 slices Canadian bacon diced (roughly 2 tablespoons)

Canola oil nonstick cooking spray, as required

⅓ cup Cheddar cheese, shredded - 3 russet potatoes, medium

⅓ cup Mozzarella cheese - salt as needed

On the Side: - Salsa & sour cream

Directions: Combine the entire Pico De Gallo ingredients together in a large bowl; mix well. When done, place in a refrigerator until ready to use.

Preheat your oven to 400 F in advance. Place potatoes in oven & bake until tender, for an hour. Set aside at room temperature until easy to handle. When done, cut them lengthwise 2 times. This should make 3 ½ to ¾" slices, throwing the middle slices away.

Increase your oven's temperature to 450 F. Take a spoon & scoop out the inside of the potato skins. Ensure that you must leave at least ¼ of an inch of the potato inside each skin. Spray the potato skin completely on all sides with the spray of nonstick canola oil. Put the skins, cut-side facing up on a large-sized cookie sheet. Sprinkle them with salt & bake in the preheated oven until the edges start to turn brown, for 12 to 15 minutes.

Combine both the cheeses together in a large bowl. Sprinkle approximately 1 ½ tablespoons of the mixture on each potato skin. Then sprinkle a teaspoon of the Canadian bacon over the cheese. Top this with a large tablespoon of the pico de gallo and then sprinkle each skin with some more of cheese.

Place the skins into the oven again & bake until the cheese melts, for 2 to 4 more minutes. Remove & let them sit for a minute. Slice each one lengthwise using a sharp knife. Serve hot with some salsa and sour cream on the side.

Nutrition: Calories: 254, Fat: 24 g, Carbs: 43 g, Protein: 55 g, Sodium: 779 mg

Applebee's Chicken Wings

Preparation Time: 15 minutes

Cooking Time: 35 minutes

Servings: 6

Ingredients:

35 chicken wings

1 ½ tablespoon flour

3 tablespoons vinegar

1 ¼ teaspoon cayenne pepper

1 tablespoon Worcestershire sauce

12 ounces Louisiana hot sauce

¼ teaspoon garlic powder

Directions:

Cook the chicken wings either by deep-frying or baking.

Mix the entire sauce ingredients (except the flour) together over low-medium heat in a large saucepan. Cook until warm and then add in the flour; stir well until you get your desired level of thickness.

When thick; cover the bottom of 9x13" baking dish with the sauce. Combine the leftover sauce with the cooked wings & place them in the baking dish. Bake until warm, for 15 to 20 minutes, at 300 F.

Serve with blue-cheese dressing and celery sticks. Enjoy.

Nutrition: Calories: 189, Fat: 11 g, Carbs: 35 g, Protein: 46 g, Sodium: 2316 g

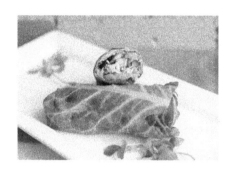

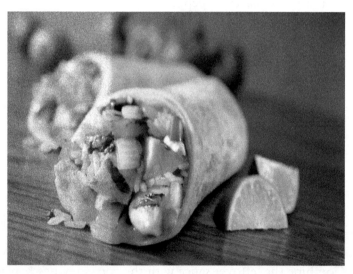

Appetizers II

Panda Express's Chicken Potstickers

Preparation Time: 40 minutes

Cooking Time: 30 minutes

Servings: 50

Ingredients:

½ cup + 2 tablespoons soy sauce, divided

1 tablespoon rice vinegar

3 tablespoons chives, divided

1 tablespoon sesame seeds

1 teaspoon sriracha hot sauce

1-pound ground pork

3 cloves garlic, minced

1 egg, beaten

1½ tablespoons sesame oil

1 tablespoon fresh ginger, minced

50 dumpling wrappers

1 cup vegetable oil, for frying

1-quart water

Directions:

In a mixing bowl, whisk together the ½ cup of soy sauce, vinegar, 1 tablespoon of the chives, sesame seeds and sriracha to make the dipping sauce.

In a separate bowl, mix together the pork, garlic, egg, the rest of the chives, the 2 tablespoons of soy sauce, sesame oil and the ginger.

Add about 1 tablespoon of the filling to each dumpling wrapper.

Pinch the sides of the wrappers together to seal. You may need to wet the edges a bit, so they'll stick.

Heat the cup of oil in a large skillet. When hot, working in batches, add the dumplings and cook until golden brown on all sides. Take care of not overloading your pan.

Add the water and cook until tender, then serve with the dipping sauce.

Nutrition: Calories: 182, Fat: 2.3 g, Carbs: 19 g, Protein: 11.2 g, Sodium: 331 g

Panda Express's Cream Cheese Rangoon

Preparation Time: 5 minutes

Cooking Time: 5 minutes

Servings: 24 minutes

Ingredients:

¼ cup green onions, chopped

½ pound cream cheese, softened

½ teaspoon garlic powder

½ teaspoon salt

24 wonton wrappers

Oil for frying

Directions:

Add the green onions, cream cheese, garlic powder and salt to a medium sized bowl and mix together.

Lay the wonton wrappers out and moisten the edges of the first one. Add about ½ tablespoon of filling to the center of the wrapper and seal by pinching the edges together, starting with the corners and working your way inward. Make sure it is sealed tightly. Repeat with the remaining wrappers.

Add about 3 inches of oil to a large pot. Heat it to about 350°F, then add the wontons a few at a time and cook until brown.

Remove from oil and place on a paper-towel-lined plate to drain.

Nutrition: Calories: 193, Fat: 5 g, Carbs: 100 g, Protein: 11 g, Sodium: 123 g

Panda Express's Chicken Egg Roll

Preparation Time: 10 minutes

Cooking Time: 5 minutes

Servings: 6-8

Ingredients:

2 tablespoons soy sauce, divided

2 cloves garlic, minced, divided - 2 green onions, chopped, divided

3 tablespoons vegetable oil, divided

½ pound boneless skinless chicken breasts, cooked whole & cut in pieces

½ head green cabbage, thinly shredded

1 large carrot, peeled and shredded - 1 cup bean sprouts

12–16 egg roll wrappers

1 tablespoon cornstarch mixed with 3 tablespoons water

Peanut Oil for frying

Directions:

In a resealable plastic bag, combine 1 tablespoon of the soy sauce with 1 clove of minced garlic, 1 green onion, and 1 tablespoon of the oil. Mix well. Add the cut-up chicken pieces, seal the bag, and squish it around to make sure the chicken is covered. Refrigerate for at least 30 minutes.

After the chicken has marinated, pour 1 tablespoon of the oil into a large skillet and heat over medium-high heat. When the oil is hot, add the chicken and cook, stirring occasionally, until the chicken is cooked through. Remove the chicken from the skillet and set aside. Pour the remaining tablespoon of oil into the skillet and add the cabbage, carrots and remaining soy sauce. Cook and stir until the carrots and cabbage start to soften, then add the bean sprouts and the remaining garlic and green onions. Cook another minute or so.

Drain the chicken and vegetables thoroughly using either a cheesecloth or a mesh strainer. Getting all the excess liquid out will keep the egg rolls from getting soggy. In a large saucepan or Dutch oven, heat 3 inches of oil to 375°F. Place about 2 tablespoons of the chicken and vegetables into the center of each egg roll wrapper. Fold the ends up and roll up to cover the filling. Seal by dipping your finger in the water and cornstarch mixture and covering the edges.

Cook the egg rolls in batches, a few at a time, for about five minutes or until golden brown and crispy. Remove from oil to a paper-towel-lined plate to drain.

Nutrition: Calories: 349, Fat: 4 g, Carbs: 176 g, Protein: 13 g, Sodium: 340 g

Panda Express's Veggie Spring Roll

Preparation Time: 15 minutes

Cooking Time: 5 minutes

Servings: 6-8

Ingredients:

4 teaspoons vegetable oil, divided

3 eggs, beaten

1 medium head cabbage, finely shredded

½ carrot, julienned

1 (8-ounce) can shredded bamboo shoots

1 cup dried, shredded wood ear mushroom, rehydrated

1-pound Chinese barbecue or roasted pork, cut into matchsticks

½ cup chopped Chinese yellow chives

1 green onion, thinly sliced

2½ teaspoons soy sauce

1 teaspoon salt

1 teaspoon sugar

1 (14-ounce) package egg roll wrappers

1 egg white, beaten

1-quart oil for frying, or as needed

Directions:

In a large skillet, heat 1 tablespoon of oil over medium-high heat.

When the skillet is hot, add the beaten eggs and cook until firm, then flip and cook a bit longer like an omelet. When set, remove from the pan. Cut into strips and set aside.

Add the remaining oil to the skillet and heat. When hot, add the cabbage and carrot and cook for a couple of minutes until they start to soften. Then add the bamboo shoots, mushrooms, pork, green onions, chives, soy sauce, salt and sugar. Cook until the veggies are soft, then stir in the egg. Transfer the mixture to a bowl and refrigerate for about 1 hour.

When cooled, add about 2-3 tablespoons of filling to each egg roll wrapper. Brush some of the beaten egg around the edges of the wrapper and roll up, tucking in the ends first.

When all of the wrappers are filled, heat about 6 inches of oil to 350°F in a deep saucepan, Dutch oven or fryer.

Add the egg rolls to the hot oil a couple at a time. When golden brown and crispy, remove from oil to a paper-towel-lined plate to drain.

Serve with chili sauce or sweet and sour sauce.

Nutrition: Calories: 132, Fat: 3.3 g, Carbs: 5.5 g, Protein:32 g, Sodium: 213 g

PF Chang's Hot and Sour Soup

Preparation Time: 10 minutes

Cooking Time: 10 minutes

Servings: 4-6

Ingredients:

6 ounces chicken breasts, cut into thin strips

1-quart chicken stock

1 cup soy sauce

1 teaspoon white pepper

1 (6 ounce) can bamboo shoots, cut into strips

6 ounces wood ear mushrooms, cut into strips or canned straw mushrooms, if wood ear can't be found

½ cup cornstarch

½ cup water

2 eggs, beaten

½ cup white vinegar

6 ounces silken tofu, cut into strips

Sliced green onions for garnish

Directions:

Cook the chicken strips in a hot skillet until cooked through. Set aside.

Add the chicken stock, soy sauce, pepper and bamboo shoots to a stockpot and bring to a boil. Stir in the chicken and let cook for about 3-4 minutes.

In a small dish, make a slurry with the cornstarch and water. Add a bit at a time to the stockpot until the broth thickens to your desired consistency.

Stir in the beaten eggs and cook for about 45 seconds or until the eggs are done.

Remove from the heat and add the vinegar and tofu.

Garnish with sliced green onions.

Nutrition: Calories: 345, Fat: 1.2 g, Carbs: 2.2 g, Protein: 23.3 g, Sodium: 145

PF Chang's Lettuce Wraps

Preparation Time: 10 minutes

Cooking Time: 10 minutes

Servings: 4

Ingredients:

1 tablespoon olive oil

1-pound ground chicken

2 cloves garlic, minced

1 onion, diced

¼ cup hoisin sauce

2 tablespoons soy sauce

1 tablespoon rice wine vinegar

1 tablespoon ginger, freshly grated

1 tablespoon Sriracha (optional)

1 (8-ounce) can whole water chestnuts, drained and diced

2 green onions, thinly sliced

Kosher salt and freshly ground black pepper to taste

1 head iceberg lettuce

Directions:

Add the oil to a deep skillet or saucepan and heat over medium-high heat. When hot, add the chicken and cook until it is completely cooked through. Stir while cooking to make sure it is properly crumbled.

Drain any excess fat from the skillet, then add the garlic, onion, hoisin sauce, soy sauce, ginger, sriracha and vinegar. Cook until the onions have softened, then stir in the water chestnuts and green onion and cook for another minute or so. Add salt and pepper to taste.

Serve with lettuce leaves and eat by wrapping them up like a taco.

Nutrition: Calories: 156, Fat: 4.3 g, Carbs: 3.7 g, Protein:27 g, Sodium: 250 g

PF Chang's Shrimp Dumplings

Preparation Time: 20 minutes

Cooking Time: 10 minutes

Servings: 4-6

Ingredients:

1 pound medium shrimp, peeled, deveined, washed and dried, divided

2 tablespoons carrot, finely minced

2 tablespoons green onion, finely minced

1 teaspoon ginger, freshly minced

2 tablespoons oyster sauce

¼ teaspoon sesame oil

1 package wonton wrappers

Sauce

1 cup soy sauce

2 tablespoons white vinegar

½ teaspoon chili paste

2 tablespoons granulated sugar

½ teaspoon ginger, freshly minced

Sesame oil to taste

1 cup water

1 tablespoon cilantro leaves

Directions:

In a food processor or blender, finely mince ½ pound of the shrimp.

Dice the other ½ pound of shrimp.

In a mixing bowl, combine both the minced and diced shrimp with the remaining ingredients.

Spoon about 1 teaspoon of the mixture into each wonton wrapper. Wet the edges of the wrapper with your finger, then fold up and seal tightly.

Cover and refrigerate for at least an hour.

In a medium bowl, combine all of the ingredients for the sauce and stir until well combined.

When ready to serve, boil water in a saucepan and cover with a steamer. You may want to lightly oil the steamer to keep the dumplings from sticking. Steam the dumplings for 7–10 minutes.

Serve with sauce.

Nutrition: Calories: 244, Fat: 20 g, Carbs: 57 g, Protein:63 g, Sodium: 354 g

PF Chang's Spicy Chicken Noodle Soup

Preparation Time: 15 minutes

Cooking Time: 15 minutes

Servings: 4-6

Ingredients:

2 quarts chicken stock

1 tablespoon granulated sugar

3 tablespoons white vinegar

2 cloves garlic, minced

1 tablespoon ginger, freshly minced

¼ cup soy sauce

Sriracha sauce to taste

Red pepper flakes to taste

1-pound boneless chicken breast, cut into thin 2-3 inch pieces

3 tablespoons cornstarch

Salt to taste

1 cup mushrooms, sliced

1 cup grape tomatoes, halved

3 green onions, sliced

2 tablespoons fresh cilantro, chopped

½ pound pasta, cooked to just under package directions and drained

Directions:

Add the chicken stock, sugar, vinegar, garlic, ginger, soy sauce, Sriracha and red pepper flakes to a large saucepan. Bring to a boil, then lower the heat to a simmer. Let cook for 5 minutes.

Season chicken with salt to taste. In a resealable bag, combine the chicken and the cornstarch. Shake to coat.

Add the chicken to the simmering broth a piece at a time. Then add the mushrooms. Continue to cook for another 5 minutes.

Stir in the tomatoes, green onions, cilantro, and cooked pasta.

Serve with additional cilantro.

Nutrition: Calories: 100, Fat: 3.7 g, Carbs: 6.7 g, Protein: 48 g Sodium: 187 g

Pei Wei 's Thai Chicken Satay

Preparation Time: 20 minutes

Cooking Time: 10-20 minutes

Marinating Time: 20 minutes

Servings: 2-4

Ingredients:

1-pound boneless, skinless chicken thighs

6-inch bamboo skewers, soaked in water

Thai satay marinade

1 tablespoon coriander seeds

1 teaspoon cumin seeds

2 teaspoons chopped lemongrass

1 teaspoon salt

1 teaspoon turmeric powder

¼ teaspoon roasted chili

½ cup coconut milk

1½ tablespoons light brown sugar

1 teaspoon lime juice

2 teaspoons fish sauce

Peanut sauce

2 tablespoons soy sauce

1 tablespoon rice wine vinegar

2 tablespoons brown sugar

¼ cup peanut butter

1 teaspoon chipotle Tabasco

Whisk all ingredients until well incorporated. Store in an airtight container in the refrigerator. Will last for 3 days.

Thai sweet cucumber relish

¼ cup white vinegar

¾ cup sugar

¾ cup water

1 tablespoon ginger, minced

1 Thai red chili, minced

1 medium cucumber

1 tablespoon toasted peanuts, chopped

Directions:

Cut any excess fat from the chicken, then cut into strips about 3 inches long and 1 inch wide. Thread the strips onto the skewers.

Prepare the Thai Satay Marinade and the Peanut Sauce in separate bowls by simply whisking together all of the ingredients for each.

Dip the chicken skewers in the Thai Satay Marinade and allow to marinate for at least 4 hours. Reserve the marinade when you remove the chicken skewers.

You can either cook the skewers on the grill, basting with the marinade halfway through, or you can do the same in a 350-degree F oven. They taste better on the grill.

To prepare the Cucumber Relish, simply add all of the ingredients together and stir to make sure the cucumber is coated.

When the chicken skewers are done cooking, serve with peanut sauce and the cucumber relish.

Nutrition: Calories: 298, Fat: 5.4 g, Carbs: 7.5 g, Protein: 61g, Sodium: 190 g

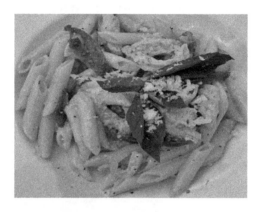

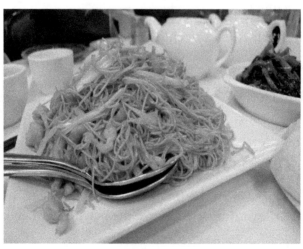

Pasta

Pesto Cavatappi from Noodles & Company

Preparation Time: 5 minutes

Cooking Time: 20 minutes

Servings: 80

Ingredients:

4 quarts water 1 tablespoon salt

1-pound macaroni pasta 1 teaspoon olive oil

1 large tomato, finely chopped

4-ounce mushrooms, finely chopped

¼ cup chicken broth ¼ cup dry white wine

¼ cup heavy cream 1 cup pesto

1 cup Parmesan cheese, grated

Directions:

Add water and salt to a pot. Bring to a boil. Put in pasta and cook for 10 minutes or until al dente. Drain and set aside.

In a pan, heat oil. Sauté tomatoes and mushrooms for 5 minutes. Pour in broth, wine, and cream. Bring to a boil. Reduce heat to medium and simmer for 2 minutes or until mixture is thick. Stir in pesto and cook for another 2 minutes. Toss in pasta. Mix until fully coated.

Transfer onto plates and sprinkle with Parmesan cheese.

Nutrition: Calories: 637, Fat: 42 g, Carbs: 48 g, Protein: 19 g, Sodium: 1730 mg

Cajun Chicken Pasta from Chili's

Preparation Time: 10 minutes

Cooking Time: 20 minutes

Servings: 4

Ingredients:

2 chicken breasts, boneless and skinless

1 tablespoon olive oil, divided

1 tablespoon Cajun seasoning

3 quarts water

½ tablespoon salt

8 ounces penne pasta

2 tablespoons unsalted butter

3 garlic cloves, minced

1 cup heavy cream

½ teaspoon lemon zest

¼ cup Parmesan cheese, shredded

Salt and black pepper, to taste

1 tablespoon oil

2 Roma tomatoes, diced

2 tablespoons parsley chopped

Directions:

Place chicken in a Ziploc bag. Add 1 tablespoon oil and Cajun seasoning. Using your hands, combine chicken and mixture until well-coated. Seal tightly and set aside to marinate.

Cook pasta in a pot filled with salt and boiling water. Follow package instructions. Drain and set aside.

In a skillet, heat butter over medium heat. Sauté garlic for 1 minute or until aromatic. Slowly add cream, followed by lemon zest. Cook for 1 minute, stirring continuously until fully blended. Toss in Parmesan cheese. Mix until sauce is a little thick, then add salt and pepper. Add pasta and combine until well-coated. Transfer onto a bowl and keep warm.

In a separate skillet, heat remaining oil. Cook chicken over medium-high heat for about 5 minutes on each side or until fully cooked through. Transfer onto chopping board and cut into thin strips.

Top pasta with chicken and sprinkle with tomatoes and parsley on top.

Serve.

Nutrition: Calories: 655, Fat: 38 g, Carbs: 47 g, Protein: 31 g, Sodium: 359 mg

Chow Mein from Panda Express

Preparation Time: 10 minutes

Cooking Time: 10 minutes

Servings: 4

Ingredients:

8 quarts water

12 ounces Yakisoba noodles

¼ cup soy sauce

3 garlic cloves, finely chopped

1 tablespoon brown sugar

2 teaspoons ginger, grated

¼ teaspoon white pepper, ground

2 tablespoons olive oil

1 onion, finely chopped

3 celery stalks, sliced on the bias

2 cups cabbage, chopped

Directions:

In a pot, bring water to a boil. Cook Yakisoba noodles for about 1 minute until noodles separate. Drain and set aside.

Combine soy sauce, garlic, brown sugar, ginger, and white pepper in a bowl.

In a pan, heat oil on medium-high heat. Sauté onion and celery for 3 minutes or until soft. Add cabbage and stir-fry for an additional minute. Mix in noodles and soy sauce mixture. Cook for 2 minutes, stirring continuously until noodles are well-coated.

Transfer into bowls. Serve.

Nutrition: Calories: 382, Fat: 8 g, Carbs: 72 g, Protein: 14 g, Sodium: 1194 mg

Rattlesnake Pasta from Pizzeria Uno

Preparation Time: 5 minutes

Cooking Time: 25 minutes

Servings: 6

Ingredients:

Pasta:

4 quarts

1-pound penne pasta

1 dash of salt

Chicken:

2 tablespoons butter

2 cloves garlic, finely chopped

½ tablespoon Italian seasoning

1-pound chicken breast, boneless and skinless, cut into small squares

Sauce:

4 tablespoons butter

2 cloves garlic, finely chopped - ¼ cup all-purpose flour

1 tablespoon - salt ¾ teaspoon white pepper

2 cups milk - 1 cup half-and-half

¾ cup Parmesan cheese, shredded

8 ounces Colby cheese, shredded

3 jalapeno peppers, chopped

Directions:

In a pot of boiling water, add salt, and cook pasta according to package instructions. Drain well and set aside.

To prepare the chicken, heat butter in a pan. Sauté garlic and Italian seasoning for 1 minute. Add chicken and cook 5-7 minutes or until cooked thoroughly, flipping halfway through. Transfer onto a plate once. Set aside.

In the same pan, prepare the sauce. Add butter and heat until melted. Stir in garlic and cook for 30 seconds. Then, add flour, salt, and pepper. Cook for 2 more minutes, stirring continuously. Pour in milk and half-and-half. Keep stirring until sauce turns thick and smooth.

Toss in chicken, jalapeno peppers, and pasta. Stir until combined.

Serve.

Nutrition: Calories: 44 g, Fat: 44 g, Carbs: 72 g, Protein: 40 g, Sodium: 1791 mg

Copycat Kung Pao Spaghetti from California Pizza Kitchen

Preparation Time: 10 minutes

Cooking Time: 20 minutes

Servings: 4

Ingredients:

1-pound spaghetti

2 tablespoons vegetable oil

3 chicken breasts, boneless and skinless

Salt and pepper, to taste

4 garlic cloves, finely chopped

½ cup dry roasted peanuts

6 green onions, cut into half-inch pieces

10-12 Dried bird eyes hot peppers

Sauce:

½ cup soy sauce

½ cup chicken broth

½ cup dry sherry

2 tablespoons red chili paste with garlic

¼ cup sugar

2 tablespoons red wine vinegar

2 tablespoons cornstarch

1 tablespoon sesame oil

Directions:

Follow instructions on package to cook spaghetti noodles. Drain and set aside.

Add oil to a large pan over medium-high heat. Generously season chicken with salt and pepper, then add to pan once hot. Cook for about 3 to 4 minutes. Turn chicken over and cook for another 3 to 4 minutes. Remove from heat and allow to cool.

Mix together all sauce ingredients in a bowl.

Once chicken is cool enough to handle, chop chicken into small pieces. Set aside.

Return pan to heat. Add garlic and sauté for about 1 minute until aromatic. Pour in prepared sauce, then stir. Once boiling, lower heat and allow to simmer for about 1 to 2 minutes or until liquid thickens. Add pasta, cooked chicken, peanuts, hot peppers, and scallions. Mix well.

Serve.

Nutrition: Calories: 548, Fat: 22 g, Saturated Fat: 7 g, Carbs: 67 g, Sugars: 16 g, Fibers: 4 g, Protein: 15 g, Sodium: 2028 mg

Three Cheese Chicken Penne from Applebee's

Preparation Time: 10 minutes

Cooking Time: 1 hour

Servings: 4

Ingredients:

2 boneless skinless chicken breasts

1 cup Italian salad dressing

3 cups penne pasta

6 tablespoons olive oil, divided

15 ounces Alfredo sauce

8 ounces combination mozzarella, Parmesan, and provolone cheeses, grated

4 roma tomatoes, seeded and diced

4 tablespoons fresh basil, diced

2 cloves garlic, finely chopped

Shredded parmesan cheese for serving

Directions:

Preheat oven to 350°F.

In a bowl, add chicken then drizzle with Italian dressing. Mix to fully coat chicken with dressing. Cover using plastic wrap and keep inside refrigerator overnight but, if you're in a hurry, at least 2 hours is fine.

Follow instructions on package to cook penne pasta. Drain, then set aside.

Brush 3 tablespoons oil onto grates of grill then preheat to medium-high heat. Add marinated chicken onto grill, discarding the marinade.

Cook chicken until both sides are fully cooked and internal temperature measures 165°F. Remove from grill. Set aside until cool enough to handle. Then, cut chicken into thin slices.

In a large bowl, add cooked noodles, Alfredo sauce, and grilled chicken. Mix until combined.

Drizzle remaining oil onto large casserole pan, then pour noodle mixture inside. Sprinkle cheeses on top. Bake for about 15-20 minutes or until cheese turns a golden and edges of mixture begins to bubble. Remove from oven.

Mix tomatoes, basil, and garlic in a bowl. Add on top of pasta.

Sprinkle parmesan cheese before serving.

Nutrition: Calories: 1402, Fat: 93 g, Saturated fat: 27 g, Carbs: 91 g, Sugar: 7 g, Fibers: 3 g, Protein: 62 g, Sodium: 5706 mg

Boston Market Mac n' Cheese

Preparation Time: 10 minutes

Cooking Time: 20 minutes

Servings: 8

Ingredients:

1 8-ounce package spiral pasta - 2 tablespoons butter

2 tablespoons all-purpose flour

1 ¾ cups whole milk

1 ¼ cups diced processed cheese like Velveeta™

¼ teaspoon dry mustard

½ teaspoon onion powder

1 teaspoon salt

Pepper, to taste

Directions:

Cook pasta according to package instructions. Drain, then set aside.

To prepare sauce make the roux with four and butter over medium-low heat in a large deep skillet. Add milk and whisk until well blended. Add cheese, mustard, salt, and pepper. Keep stirring until smooth.

Once pasta is cooked, transfer to a serving bowl. Pour cheese mixture on top. Toss to combine.

Serve warm.

Nutrition: Calories: 319, Fat: 17 g, Saturated Fat: 10 g, Carbs: 28 g, Sugar: 7 g, Fibers: 1 g, Protein: 17 g, Sodium: 1134 mg

Macaroni Grill's Pasta Milano

Preparation Time: 5 minutes

Cooking Time: 20 minutes

Servings: 6

Ingredients:

1 pound bowtie pasta

2 teaspoons olive oil

1 pound chicken, chopped into small pieces

1 12-ounce package mushrooms, chopped

1 cup onion, minced

2 garlic cloves, finely minced

½ cup sun dried tomatoes, diced

1½ cups half and half

1 tablespoon butter, softened

½ cup Parmesan cheese, shredded, plus some more for serving

1 teaspoon black pepper, ground

1 tablespoon fresh basil, minced

Directions:

Follow instructions on package to cook bowtie pasta. Drain, then set aside.

Add oil to a pan over medium-high heat. Once hot, add chicken and stir-fry for about 5 to 6 minutes until cooked through. Set chicken aside onto a plate.

In the same pan, toss in mushrooms, onions, garlic, and sundried tomatoes. Sauté until onions turn soft and mushrooms become a light brown, then sprinkle salt and pepper to season. Return chicken to pan and mix.

Mix half and half, butter, Parmesan, pepper, and basil in a small bowl.

Add half and half mixture to pan. Stir, and let simmer for about 3 to 4 minutes or until pan ingredients are thoroughly heated. Mix in pasta until coated well.

Serve.

Nutrition: Calories: 600, Fat: 18 g, Saturated Fat: 9 g, Carbs: 69 g, Sugar: 8 g, Fibers: 5 g, Protein: 42 g, Sodium: 349 mg

Olive Garden's Fettuccine Alfredo

Preparation Time: 5 minutes

Cooking Time: 25 minutes

Servings: 6

Ingredients:

½ cup butter, melted

2 tablespoons cream cheese

1 pint heavy cream 1 teaspoon garlic powder

Some salt

Some black pepper

⅔ cup parmesan cheese, grated

1 pound fettuccine, cooked

Directions:

Melt the cream cheese in the melted butter over medium heat until soft.

Add the heavy cream and season the mixture with garlic powder, salt, and pepper.

Reduce the heat to low and allow the mixture to simmer for another 15 to 20 minutes.

Remove the mixture from heat and add in the parmesan. Stir everything to melt the cheese.

Pour the sauce over the pasta and serve.

Nutrition: Calories: 767.3, Fat: 52.9 g, Carbs: 57.4 g, Protein: 17.2 g, Sodium: 367 mg

Red Lobster's Shrimp Pasta

Preparation Time: 5 minutes

Cooking Time: 30 minutes

Servings: 4

Ingredients:

8 ounces linguini or spaghetti pasta

⅓ cup extra virgin olive oil

3 garlic cloves

1 pound shrimp, peeled, deveined

⅔ cup clam juice or chicken broth

⅓ cup white wine

1 cup heavy cream

½ cup parmesan cheese, freshly grated

¼ teaspoon dried basil, crushed

¼ teaspoon dried oregano, crushed

Fresh parsley and parmesan cheese for garnish

Directions:

Cook the Pasta according to package directions.

Simmer the garlic in hot oil over low heat, until tender.

Increase the heat to low to medium and add the shrimp. When the shrimp is cooked, transfer it to a separate bowl along with the garlic. Keep the remaining oil in the pan.

Pour the clam or chicken broth into the pan and bring to a boil.

Add the wine and adjust the heat to medium. Keep cooking the mixture for another 3 minutes.

While stirring the mixture, reduce the heat to low and add in the cream and cheese. Keep stirring.

When the mixture thickens, return the shrimp to the pan and throw in the remaining ingredients (except the pasta).

Place the pasta in a bowl and pour the sauce over it.

Mix everything together and serve. Garnish with parsley and parmesan cheese, if desired

Nutrition: Calories: 590, Fat: 26 g, Carbs: 54 g, Protein: 34 g, Sodium: 1500 mg

+ Cheesecake Factory's Cajun Jambalaya Pasta

Preparation Time: 10 minutes

Cooking Time: 40 minutes

Servings: 4

Ingredients:

Cajun Seasoning Blend:

1 teaspoon white pepper

1 teaspoon cayenne pepper

3 teaspoons salt

1 teaspoon paprika

½ teaspoon garlic powder

½ teaspoon onion powder

Chicken and Shrimp:

2 boneless skinless chicken breasts, halved, cut into bite-size pieces

½ pound large shrimp, peeled, deveined

1 tablespoon olive oil

Pasta:

5 quarts water

6 ounces fettuccine

6 ounces spinach fettuccine

Jambalaya:

1 tablespoon olive oil

2 medium tomatoes, chopped

1 medium onion, sliced

1 green bell pepper, sliced

1 red bell pepper, sliced

1 yellow bell pepper, sliced

1½ cups chicken stock

1 tablespoon cornstarch

2 tablespoons white wine

2 teaspoons arrowroot powder

2 teaspoons fresh parsley, chopped

Directions:

Mix all of the Cajun seasoning blend ingredients together to make the seasoning. Divide the seasoning into 3 equal parts.

Coat the chicken and shrimp with ⅓ of the seasoning each.

Cook pasta according to package directions.

While waiting for the pasta, sauté the spiced chicken in heated oil in a large skillet.

When the chicken starts turning brown, stir in the shrimp and cook until the chicken is cooked tough and shrimp turn pink.

Transfer the chicken and shrimp to a plate and set aside.

Using the same pan, warm the oil for the jambalaya over medium heat. Add the tomatoes, onions, peppers, and remaining 1/3 of the seasoning mix. Sauté for 10 minutes.

When the vegetables turn brownish-black, add the chicken and shrimp back to the mix.

Pour in ¾ cup of the chicken stock to deglaze the pan. Gently scrape the pan to remove the burnt particles. Turn the heat to high and allow the mixture to cook.

When the broth has evaporated completely, add in the remaining stock and cook for another 5 minutes.

Turn the heat down to low and leave the mixture to rest over heat. In a bowl, mix the white wine and arrowroot until it dissolves.

Add the mixture to the jambalaya. Turn the heat to low and leave the mixture to simmer.

When the jambalaya and pasta are done, assemble the dish by:

a) Putting the pasta as the first layer;

b) Covering the pasta with the jambalaya sauce; and

c) Garnish each plate with parsley.

Nutrition: Calories: 563.9, Fat: 13.3 g, Carbs: 73.8 g, Protein: 35.9 g, Sodium: 1457.6 mg

Olive Garden's Steak Gorgonzola

Preparation Time: 10 minutes

Cooking Time: 1 hour and 30 minutes

Servings: 6

Ingredients:

Pasta:

2½ pounds boneless beef top sirloin steaks, cut into ½-inch cubes

1 pound fettucine or linguini, cooked

2 tablespoons sun-dried tomatoes, chopped

2 tablespoons balsamic vinegar glaze

Some fresh parsley leaves, chopped

Marinade:

1½ cups Italian dressing

1 tablespoon fresh rosemary, chopped

1 tablespoon fresh lemon juice (optional)

Spinach Gorgonzola Sauce:

4 cups baby spinach, trimmed

2 cups Alfredo sauce (recipe follows)

½ cup green onion, chopped

6 tablespoons gorgonzola, crumbled, and divided)

Directions:

Cook the pasta and set aside. Mix together the marinade ingredients in a sealable container.

Marinate the beef in the container for an hour.

While the beef is marinating, make the Spinach Gorgonzola sauce. Heat the Alfredo sauce in a saucepan over medium heat. Add spinach and green onions. Let simmer until the spinach wilt. Crumble 4 tablespoons of the Gorgonzola cheese on top of the sauce. Let melt and stir. Set aside remaining 2 tablespoons of the cheese for garnish. Set aside and cover with lid to keep warm.

When the beef is done marinating, grill each piece depending on your preference.

Toss the cooked pasta and the Alfredo sauce in a saucepan, and then transfer to a plate.

Top the pasta with the beef, and garnish with balsamic glaze, sun-dried tomatoes, crumble gorgonzola cheese, and parsley leaves.

Serve and enjoy.

Nutrition: Calories: 740.5, Fat: 27.7 g, Carbs: 66 g, Protein: 54.3 g, Sodium: 848.1 mg

+ Noodles and Company's Pad Thai

Preparation Time: 5 minutes

Cooking Time: 20 minutes

Servings: 4

Ingredients:

Sauce:

½ cup boiling water

¼ cup brown sugar

6 tablespoons lime juice

¼ cup rice vinegar

¼ cup Thai fish sauce

2 teaspoons Sriracha

Pad Thai:

12 ounces fettuccine or linguine (uncooked)

2 tablespoons canola oil, divided

½ yellow onion, sliced

3 cloves fresh garlic. pressed or minced

3 eggs, lightly beaten

½ cup cabbage, sliced

½ cup mushrooms, sliced

1 cup carrots, sliced

1 cup broccoli, chopped

Garnish: cilantro, sliced green onions, lime wedges

Directions:

Dissolve the sugar in the boiling water. When the sugar has completely dissolved, mix in the lime juice, vinegar, fish sauce, and Sriracha.

Cook the noodles.

Sauté the onion in 1 tablespoon of oil over medium to high heat for 1 minute. Add in the garlic and sauté for another 30 seconds. Mix the eggs into the garlic and onion mixture, and continue to cook until the egg is cooked completely.

Transfer the egg mixture to a bowl and add the remaining oil to the same pan. Sauté the vegetables.

When the vegetables are crispy, add in half of the sauce and cook for 1 to 3 minutes. When your desired consistency is reached, add in the egg mixture and noodles and transfer to a plate to serve.

Nutrition: Calories: 830, Fat: 18 g, Carbs: 151 g, Protein: 15 g, Sodium: 1300 mg

Cheesecake Factory's Pasta di Vinci

Preparation Time: 10 minutes

Cooking Time: 50 minutes

Servings: 4

Ingredients:

½ red onion, chopped

1 cup mushrooms, quartered

2 teaspoons garlic, chopped

1 pound chicken breast, cut into bite-size pieces

3 tablespoons butter, divided

2 tablespoons flour

2 teaspoons salt

¼ cup white wine

1 cup cream of chicken soup mixed with some milk

4 tablespoons heavy cream

Basil leaves for serving, chopped

Parmesan cheese for serving

1 pound penne pasta, cooked, drained

Directions:

Sauté the onion, mushrooms and garlic in 1 tablespoon of the butter.

When they are tender, remove them from the butter and place in a bowl. Cook the chicken in the same pan.

When the chicken is done, transfer it to the bowl containing the garlic, onions, and mushrooms, and set everything aside.

Using the same pan, make a roux using the flour and remaining butter over low to medium heat. When the roux is ready, mix in the salt, wine, and cream of chicken mixture. Continue stirring the mixture, making sure that it does not burn.

When the mixture thickens and allow the mixture to simmer for a few more minutes.

Mix in the ingredients that you set aside, and transfer the cooked pasta to a bowl or plate.

Pour the sauce over the pasta, garnish with parmesan cheese and basil, and serve.

Nutrition: Calories: 844.9, Fat: 35.8 g, Carbs: 96.5 g, Protein: 33.9 g, Sodium: 1400.2 mg

Longhorn Steakhouse's Mac & Cheese

Preparation Time: 20 minutes

Cooking Time: 20 minutes

Servings: 10

Ingredients:

1 pound cavatappi pasta, cooked

2 tablespoons butter

2 tablespoons flour

2 cups half-and-half

2 ounces gruyere cheese, shredded

8 ounces white cheddar, shredded

2 tablespoons parmesan cheese, shredded

4 ounces fontina cheese, shredded

1 teaspoon smoked paprika

4 pieces bacon, crispy, crumbled

½ cup panko bread crumbs

Directions:

Make a roux by cooking the melted butter and flour over medium heat.

When the roux is cooked, add in the half-and-half ½ cup at a time, adding more as the sauce thickens.

Slowly add the rest of the ingredients (except the pasta) one at a time, really allowing each ingredient to incorporate itself into the sauce. Continue stirring the mixture until everything is heated.

Place the pasta in a greased 13×9 baking pan or 6 individual baking dishes and pour the sauce over it. Sprinkle the bacon and panko bread crumbs over the top of the pasta.

Bake the pasta in an oven preheated to 350°F for 20-25 minutes, or until breadcrumbs start to become golden brown.

Let the pasta cool, and serve.

Nutrition: Calories: 610, Fat: 37 g, Carbs: 43 g, Protein: 26 g, Sodium: 1210 mg

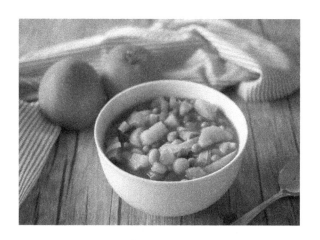

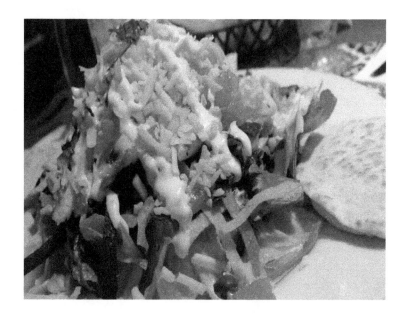

82

Soups and Side Dishes

Breadsticks

Preparation Time: 60 minutes

Cooking Time: 15 minutes

Servings: 16

Ingredients:

Breadsticks

1½ cups warm water

2 tablespoons sugar

1 packet (1 tablespoon/¾ ounce) yeast

2 teaspoons fine sea salt (and a bit extra to sprinkle on top)

2 tablespoons butter, softened

4-5 cups bread flour (you can also use all-purpose flour, but the breadsticks will turn out denser)

Topping

¼ cup butter

1 teaspoon garlic powder

Directions:

To make the breadsticks, combine the warm water, sugar, and yeast in a large bowl.

Proof for 10 minutes. Mix in the salt, softened butter, and 3 cups of bread flour.

Mix in the rest of the bread flour to get a soft dough.

Cover the bowl with a damp towel and set aside in a warm place. Let dough rise for 1 hour.

Gently knead the dough and separate into 14–16 balls.

Roll each ball into a log of your desired length. Place on two cookie sheets and let rise for 15–30 minutes.

To make the topping, melt the butter and mix with the garlic powder.

Brush the topping mixture over the breadsticks and finish with sprinkles of sea salt.

Bake at 400°F for 12–14 minutes.

Brush the remaining garlic butter on top of the breadsticks.

Nutrition: Calories: 156, Fat: 67 g, Carbs: 98. 7 g, Protein: 34 .9 g, Sodium: 756 mg

Chicken Gnocchi Soup

Preparation Time: 10 minutes

Cooking Time: 8 minutes

Servings: 4

Ingredients:

1 tablespoon oil

1½ pounds chicken breast, cubed

½ cup celery, chopped

½ cup onion, chopped

2 cups chicken broth

1 cup matchstick carrots

1 teaspoon thyme

3 cups half and half

1 (16-ounce) package gnocchi

2 cups fresh spinach

Directions:

Place oil, chicken, and celery in the Instant Pot. Sauté until meat is brown.

Mix in chicken broth, carrots, and thyme. Close the lid and the pressure release valve.

Set to Manual, High Pressure for 4 minutes. Once completed, quick release pressure.

Open the lid and set to sauté. Add spinach, half and half and gnocchi. Leave Instant Pot on sauté to heat the soup until it is boiling.

Let boil and keep stirring for 3 minutes or until gnocchi is cooked. Serve.

Nutrition: Calories: 237 Fat: 45 g Carbs: 12. 7 g Protein: 45. 6 g Sodium: 458 mg

Zuppa Toscana

Preparation Time: 20 minutes

Cooking Time: 4 hours

Servings: 8

Ingredients:

1 pound ground hot Italian sausage

1 tablespoon garlic, minced

1 yellow onion, chopped

4 russet potatoes, diced

1 quart chicken broth

1 bunch kale

¾ cup heavy whipping cream

¼ cup parmesan, shredded

Directions:

In a large skillet, crumble the Italian sausage and cook on medium-high heat for about 5–8 minutes.

Add the onions and garlic and cook for about 2–3 minutes.

Drain the grease and move the cooked sausages and veggies to a 6-quart crock pot (or larger). Add the diced potatoes and season with salt and pepper.

Pour in enough chicken broth to cover the potatoes. Add up to 2 cups of water if there isn't enough chicken broth.

Stir, then cover. Set to cook on low for 5–6 hours or high for 3–4 hours.

Add the kale and heavy whipping cream. Stir

Replace the cover and let cook for another 30 minutes on high. Serve topped with parmesan cheese.

Nutrition: Calories: 345, Fat: 87 g, Carbs: 83. 9 g, Protein: 69. 2 g, Sodium: 837 mg

Minestrone

Preparation Time: 15 minutes

Cooking Time: 1 hour and 20 minutes

Servings: 6 to 8

Ingredients:

3 tablespoons olive oil

1 medium onion, diced

1 small zucchini, chopped

1 (14-ounce) can Italian-style green beans

1 stalk celery, diced

4 teaspoons garlic, minced

1 quart vegetable broth

2 (15-ounce) cans red kidney beans, drained

2 (15-ounce) cans great northern beans, drained

1 (14-ounce) can diced tomatoes with juice

½ cup carrot, shredded

½ cup dry red wine (optional) ½ cup tomato paste

1 teaspoon oregano   1 teaspoon basil

¼ teaspoon thyme

½ teaspoon garlic powder

½ teaspoon onion powder   1 bay leaf

3 cups hot water

4 cups fresh spinach

1½ cups shell pasta

Salt and pepper to taste

Directions:

In a large stockpot, heat olive oil and sauté onion, celery, zucchini and carrots over medium heat.

Stir in garlic, green beans, and tomato paste. Then add broth, red wine, hot water, tomatoes, green beans, oregano, basil, thyme, garlic powder, onion powder, and bay leaf.

Bring soup to a boil. Reduce heat, cover and simmer for 45 minutes. Remove bay leaf.

Mix in spinach and pasta. Cook for 30 minutes. Serve.

Nutrition: Calories: 265, Fat: 45 g, Carbs: 32.4 g, Protein: 54.8 g, Sodium: 3457 mg

House Salad and Dressing

Preparation Time: 10 minutes

Cooking Time: 0

Servings: 12

Ingredients:

Salad

1 head iceberg lettuce

¼ small red onion, sliced thin

6–12 black olives, pitted

6 pepperoncini

2 small roma tomatoes, sliced

Croutons

¼ cup shredded or grated romano or parmesan cheese

Dressing

1 packet Italian dressing mix

¾ cup vegetable/canola oil

¼ cup olive oil

1 tablespoon mayonnaise

⅓ cup white vinegar

¼ cup water

½ teaspoon sugar

½ teaspoon dried Italian seasoning

½ teaspoon salt

¼ teaspoon pepper

¼ teaspoon garlic powder

Directions:

To make the dressing, combine all ingredients in a small bowl. Thoroughly whisk together. Refrigerate for 1 hour to marinate.

Add the salad ingredient to a salad bowl. When ready to serve, add some of the dressing to the salad and toss to coat. Add grated cheese as a garnish as desired.

Store remaining dressing in an airtight container. Keep refrigerated and it can be stored for up to 3 weeks.

Nutrition: Calories: 435, Fat: 54. 8 g, Carbs: 46.4 g, Protein: 13.9 g, Sodium: 5675 mg

Santa Fe Crispers Salad

Preparation Time: 10 minutes

Cooking Time: 30 minutes

Servings: 4

Ingredients:

1 ½ pounds boneless skinless chicken breasts

1 tablespoon fresh cilantro, chopped

¾ cup Lawry's Santa Fe Chili Marinated with Lime and Garlic, divided

1 package (10 ounces) torn romaine lettuce, approximately 8 cups

2 tablespoons milk   1 cup black beans, drained and rinsed

½ cup sour cream   1 cup drained canned whole kernel corn

¼ cup red onion, chopped

1 medium avocado, cut into chunks

½ cup Monterey Jack, shredded

1 medium tomato, cut into chunks

Directions:

Place chicken in a large glass dish or re-sealable marinade plastic bag

Add approximately ½ cup of the Santa Fe marinade, turn several times until nicely coated

Refrigerate for 30 minutes or longer

Removed the chicken from marinade; get rid of the leftover marinade

Grill the chicken until cooked through, for 6 to 7 minutes per side, over medium heat; brushing with 2 tablespoons of the leftover marinade

Cut the chicken into thin slices.

Combine the sour cream together with milk, leftover marinade and cilantro with wire whisk in medium-sized bowl until smooth

Arrange lettuce on large serving platter

Top with the chicken, avocado, corn, beans, cheese, tomato and onion.

Serve with tortilla chips and dressing. Enjoy.

Nutrition: Calories: 676, Fat: 86 g, Carbs: 67 g, Protein: 46 g, Sodium: 2434 mg

Quesadilla Explosion Salad

Preparation Time: 20 minutes

Cooking Time: 20 minutes

Servings: 1

Ingredients:

1 vegetarian chicken patty

6 ounces bagged salad mix

For Chipotle Ranch Dressing:

1 cup 2% milk

1 packet ranch dressing mix

1 teaspoon chipotle peppers in adobo sauce

1 cup non-fat Greek yogurt

For Citrus Balsamic Vinaigrette

2 tablespoon balsamic vinegar

½ teaspoon orange zest

2 tablespoon Splenda

¼ cup orange juice

A pinch of nutmeg

For Sweet Potato Strips:

¼ medium sweet potato, washed, thinly sliced & cut into strips

nonstick cooking spray

¼ teaspoon salt

For Cheese Quesadilla:

1 mission carb balance whole wheat fajita sized tortilla

1 ounce reduced-fat Colby jack cheese, shredded

For Roasted Corn and Black Bean Salsa:

1 cup black beans, rinsed

2 ears of corn, roasted, kernels removed from cob

½ cup fresh cilantro, chopped

1 tablespoon lime juice, freshly squeezed

¼ red onion, chopped

1 jalapeno pepper, roasted, peeled, seeded, de-veined & chopped

Salt to taste

1 red bell pepper, medium, roasted, peeled, seeded & chopped

Directions:

For Sweet Potato Strips:

Preheat oven to 350 F. Lightly coat the strips with nonstick cooking spray and then, dust them lightly with the salt. Place on a large-sized cookie sheet in a single layer & bake for 15 to 20 minutes. Don't forget to stir the strips & turn halfway during the baking process.

Set aside and let cool until ready to use.

For Roasted Corn Salsa:

Add corn together with peppers & black beans to a large bowl and then squeeze the lime juice on top; add salt to taste. Give the ingredients a good stir & add the fresh cilantro.

For Chipotle Ranch Dressing:

Add yogurt and milk to the ranch dressing mix. Stir in the chipotle & store in a refrigerator.

For Citrus Balsamic Vinaigrette:

Over low heat in a large saucepan; place the entire ingredients together & cook for a minute. Set aside and let cool then refrigerate.

For Quesadilla:

1.Place the cheese on half of the tortilla & then fold over.

Lightly coat the tortilla with the nonstick cooking spray & then cook over medium-high heat in a large pan. Cook until the cheese is completely melted, for a minute per side. Cut into 4 wedges.

Prepare the veggie "chicken" patty as per the directions mentioned on the package & then slice into thin strips.

Place approximately 6 ounces of the salad mix on the plate and then top with the "chicken" strips, black bean salsa, sweet potato strips & roasted corn.

Place the cut quesadilla around the edge of the plate and then drizzle the salad with the prepared dressings.

Nutrition: Calories: 245, Fat: 59.8 g, Carbs: 67.3 g, Protein: 12. 8 g, Sodium: 4354 mg

Caribbean Shrimp Salad

Preparation Time: 20 minutes

Cooking Time: 55 minutes

Servings: 4

Ingredients:

8 cups baby spinach, fresh

¼ cup lime juice, freshly squeezed

2 tablespoons chili garlic sauce

½ teaspoon paprika

4 cups cooked shrimp, chopped (approximately 1 ½ pounds)

1 tablespoon grated lime rind

5 tablespoons seasoned rice vinegar, divided

½ teaspoon ground cumin

1 cup peeled mango, chopped

½ cup green onions, thinly sliced

2 garlic cloves, minced

1 cup radishes, julienne-cut

¼ cup peeled avocado, diced

2 tablespoons pumpkinseed kernels, unsalted

1 ½ tablespoons olive oil

Dash of salt

Directions:

In a large bowl; combine the cooked shrimp together with chili garlic sauce & 2 tablespoons of vinegar; toss well. Cover & let chill for an hour.

Now, in a small bowl; combine the leftover vinegar together with garlic cloves, oil, lime juice, lime rind, ground cumin, paprika & salt; stirring well with a whisk.

Place 2 cups of spinach on each of 4 plates; top each serving with a cup of the prepared shrimp mixture. Arrange ¼ cup radishes, ¼ cup mango & 1 tablespoon of the avocado around the shrimp on each plate. Top each serving with approximately 1 ½ teaspoons of pumpkinseed kernels & 2 tablespoons of green onions. Drizzle each salad with approximately 2 tablespoons of the vinaigrette. Serve and enjoy.

Nutrition: Calories: 124, Fat: 76.9 g, Carbs: 67. 9 g, Protein: 45. 8 g, Sodium: 568 mg

Southwest Caesar Salad

Preparation Time: 10 minutes

Cooking Time: 20 minutes

Servings: 6

Ingredients:

2 tablespoon mayonnaise

¼ teaspoon cayenne or ground red pepper

6 cups fresh romaine lettuce, washed, shredded (approximately 1 head)

⅓ cup parmesan cheese, grated

1 cup croutons

½ of a red bell pepper, cut into thin strips

1 cup whole kernel corn, frozen & thawed

½ cup fresh cilantro, chopped

2 tablespoon green onion, chopped

¼ cup olive oil

2 tablespoon lime juice, freshly squeezed

1/8 teaspoon salt

Directions:

Place onions together with mayo, ground red pepper, lime juice and salt in a blender or food processor; cover & process until blended well. Slowly add the oil at top using the feed tube & continue to process after each addition until blended well.

Toss the lettuce with the corn, croutons, bell peppers, cheese and cilantro in a large bowl.

Add the mayo mixture; evenly toss until nicely coated. Serve immediately & enjoy.

Nutrition: Calories: 265, Fat: 62 g, Carbs: 98 g, Protein: 47 g, Sodium:467 mg

Chili's Chili

Preparation Time: 10 minutes

Cooking Time: 1 hour and 10 minutes

Servings: 8

Ingredients:

For Chili:

4 pounds ground chuck - ground for chili

1 ½ cups yellow onions, chopped

16 ounces tomato sauce

1 tablespoon cooking oil

3 ¼ plus 1 cups water

1 tablespoon masa harina

For Chili Spice Blend:

1 tablespoon paprika

½ cup chili powder

1 teaspoon ground black pepper

1/8 cup ground cumin

1 teaspoon cayenne pepper or to taste

1/8 cup salt

1 teaspoon garlic powder

Directions:

Combine the entire chili spice ingredients together in a small bowl; continue to combine until thoroughly mixed.

Now, over moderate heat in a 6-quart stock pot; place & cook the meat until browned; drain. In the meantime; combine the chili spice mix together with tomato sauce & 3 ¼ cups of water in the bowl; give the ingredients a good stir until blended well.

Add the chili seasoning liquid to the browned meat; give it a good stir & bring the mixture to a boil over moderate heat.

Over medium heat in a large skillet; heat 1 tablespoon of the cooking oil & sauté the onions until translucent, for a couple of minutes. Add the sautéed onions to the chili.

Decrease the heat to low & let simmer for an hour, stirring after every 10 to 15 minutes. Combine the masa harina with the leftover water in a separate bowl; mix well. Add to the chili stock pot & cook for 10 more minutes.

Nutrition: Calories: 143, Fat: 51. 3 g, Carbs: 63.6 g, Protein: 13.8 g, Sodium: 1367 mg

Chicken Enchilada Soup

Preparation Time: 10 minutes

Cooking Time: 15 minutes

Servings: 10

Ingredients:

2 rotisserie chickens or 3 pounds cooked diced chicken

½ pound processed American cheese; cut in small cubes

3 cups yellow onions, diced

¼ cup chicken base

2 cups masa harina

½ teaspoon cayenne pepper

2 teaspoon granulated garlic

1 - 2 teaspoons salt or to taste

2 cups tomatoes, crushed

½ cup vegetable oil

2 teaspoon chili powder

4 quarts water

2 teaspoon ground cumin

Directions:

Over moderate heat in a large pot; combine oil together with onions, chicken base, granulated garlic, chili powder, cumin, cayenne & salt. Cook for 3 to 5 minutes, until onions are soft & turn translucent, stirring occasionally.

Combine 1 quart of water with masa harina in a large measuring cup or pitcher.

Continue to stir until no lumps remain. Add to the onions; bring the mixture to a boil, over moderate heat.

Once done, cook for a couple of minutes, stirring constantly. Stir in the tomatoes & leftover 3 quarts of water. Bring the soup to a boil again, stirring every now and then. Add in the cheese.

Cook until the cheese is completely melted, stirring occasionally. Add the chicken & cook until heated through. Serve immediately & enjoy.

Nutrition: Calories: 356, Fat: 53.9 g, Carbs: 25. 6 g, Protein: 12.8 g, Sodium: 454 mg

Chicken Mushroom Soup

Preparation Time: 10 minutes

Cooking Time: 4 hours and 10 minutes

Servings: 4

Ingredients:

½ cup All-purpose flour

5 boneless & skinless chicken breasts, cubed

½ small onion, diced

3 cups mushrooms, sliced

¼ cup carrots, diced

6 cups chicken Broth

¼ cup softened butter, at room temperature

3 cups heavy cream

½ teaspoon white pepper

1 teaspoon lemon juice, freshly squeezed

¼ teaspoon dried thyme

Ground black pepper & kosher salt, to taste

⅛ teaspoon dried tarragon

Directions:

Over medium heat in a large pot; heat the butter until completely melted and then toss in the onion, chicken, mushrooms & carrots. Sauté until the chicken is cooked through; cover the ingredients with the all-purpose flour.

Pour in the chicken broth, white pepper, thyme, tarragon, pepper & salt. Bring the mixture to a simmer & cook for 10 to 12 minutes.

Add the lemon juice and heavy cream. Let simmer again for 10 to 12 more minutes.

Serve hot & enjoy.

Nutrition: Calories: 146, Fat: 16.9 g, Carbs: 25.8, Protein: 41 g, Sodium: 215 mg

Carrabba's Sausage and Lentil Soup

Preparation Time: 10 minutes

Cooking Time: 1 hour 5 minutes

Servings: 6

Ingredients:

1 pound Italian sausages

1 large onion, diced

1 stalk celery, diced

2 large carrots, diced

1 small zucchini, diced

6 cups low sodium chicken broth

2 cans (14.5 ounces each) tomatoes, diced, with juice

2 cups dry lentils

2-3 garlic cloves, minced

1 ½ teaspoons salt

1 teaspoon black pepper

1-3 pinches red pepper flakes, more if you like it spicier

1 teaspoon dry basil

½ teaspoon dry oregano

½ teaspoon parsley

½ teaspoon dry thyme

Parmesan cheese for garnishing

Directions:

Preheat the oven to 350°F. Place sausages on a baking dish and poke a few holes in each sausage with a fork. Bake for 20-30 minutes, or until the sausages are done. Let cool down and slice the sausages.

Chop and mince the ingredients as specified in the ingredients list.

Place all the ingredients, except the parmesan cheese, in a large pot.

Bring the soup to a boil, then lower the heat and cover the pot.

Let the mixture simmer for an hour, adding water to reduce thickness when necessary. If you want a thicker soup, puree a portion of the soup and return it.

Ladle the soup into bowls and garnish with parmesan cheese before serving

Nutrition: Calories: 221, Fat: 10 g, Carbs: 20 g, Protein: 13 g, Sodium: 1182 mg

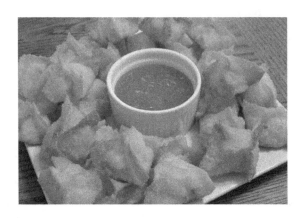

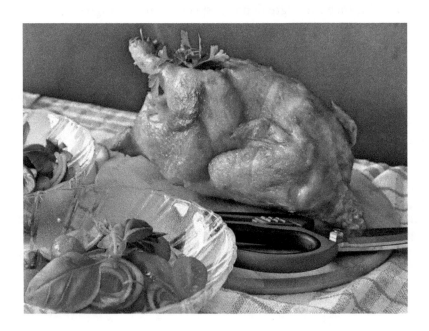

Compilation of Famous Main Dishes I

Bistro Shrimp Pasta

Preparation Time: 30 minutes

Cooking Time: 45 minutes

Servings: 8

Ingredients:

2 tablespoons olive oil

1 cup button mushrooms, quartered

1 cup grape tomatoes, halved

1 pound thin spaghetti, cooked

For the Lemon Basil Cream Sauce

¼ cup butter

4 garlic cloves, minced

2 cups heavy whipping cream

2 cups chicken broth

½ cup lemon juice

¼ cup cornstarch

½ teaspoon pepper

1 cup chopped fresh basil

For the shrimp

1 pound raw shrimp, deveined and with shells removed

2 eggs, beaten

1 cup flour

1 cup panko

1 teaspoon garlic powder

1 teaspoon Italian seasoning

3 tablespoons butter

Directions:

In a small skillet, cook the mushrooms in 2 tablespoons of olive oil. When they are soft, stir in the tomatoes and set the skillet aside.

Make the cream sauce: in a large skillet, melt the butter. Add the garlic and cook until fragrant. Pour in the cream and chicken broth, and bring to a low boil. Reduce the heat and let the sauce cook until the liquid reduces by half.

In a small dish, whisk the corn starch into the lemon juice, mixing until it is smooth and free of lumps, making slurry. Add the slurry into the chicken broth mixture.

To make the shrimp, beat the eggs in one small dish and combine the panko, flour, garlic powder, and Italian seasoning in a different one. Then dip each shrimp in the egg mixture and then into the panko.

Using the skillet you cooked the mushroom and tomatoes in, melt the 3 tablespoons of butter. When the shrimp turns nicely golden, remove it from skillet and let it drain on a plated lined with paper towel.

Add the fresh basil to the sauce and stir.

To serve, put some pasta on the plate, cover with sauce, and top with shrimp.

Nutrition: Calories: 234 Fat: 16 g Carbs: 81.9 g Protein: 76. 7 g Sodium: 656 mg

Crispy Crab Wontons

Preparation Time: 10 minutes

Cooking Time: 15 minutes

Servings: 4

Ingredients:

4 ounces cream cheese

2 tablespoons sweet and sour chili sauce (plus more for serving)

1 ½ teaspoons mustard

1 teaspoon chili garlic paste

1 teaspoon lemon juice

½ teaspoon granulated sugar

4 ounces crab meat

2 ounces sliced water chestnuts, minced

2 tablespoons green onions, finely chopped

1 ounce mozzarella cheese, grated

1 ounce fontina cheese, grated

¼ cup panko breadcrumbs

25 small square wonton wrappers, approximately 3-½ inches

Oil for frying

Directions:

In a large bowl, mix together the cream cheese, sweet and sour sauce, mustard, garlic paste, lemon juice, and sugar. Stir until well combined, then gently add in the crab, the water chestnuts, and green onions.

In a separate bowl, combine the mozzarella, fontina, and panko breadcrumbs. Carefully fold them into the cream cheese mixture, until well distributed.

Heat enough oil in a large skillet or saucepan so that the wontons won't touch the bottom when you cook them.

Lay out a wonton wrapper and fill it with about a teaspoon of filling. Pinch the sides of the wonton up and seal with a bit of water on your fingers.

When the oil is about 350°F, fry the wontons until they turn a golden brown. Transfer them to a plate lined with paper towel to drain.

Serve the wontons with sweet and sour chili sauce.

Nutrition: Calories: 724, Fat: 39 g, Carbs: 89 g, Protein: 65 g, Sodium: 1587 mg

Chicken Casserole

Preparation Time: 10 minutes

Cooking Time: 1 hour and 20 minutes

Servings: 4

Ingredients:

Crust

1 cup yellow cornmeal

⅓ cup all-purpose flour

1½ teaspoons baking powder

1 tablespoon sugar

½ teaspoon salt

½ teaspoon baking soda

2 tablespoons vegetable oil

¾ cup buttermilk

1 egg

Filling

2½ cups cooked chicken breast, cut into bite sized pieces

¼ cup chopped yellow onion

½ cup sliced celery

1 teaspoon salt

¼ teaspoon ground pepper

1 (10.5-ounce) can condensed cream of chicken soup

1¾ cups chicken broth

2 tablespoons butter

½ cup melted butter

Directions:

Preheat the oven to 375°F.

To make the crust, in a large bowl, combine all of the crust ingredients until smooth.

Dump this mixture into a buttered or greased 8×8-inch baking dish. Bake for about 20 minutes, then remove from oven and allow to cool. Reduce oven temperature to 350°F.

Crumble the cooled cornbread mixture. Add to a large mixing bowl along with ½ cup of melted butter. Set aside.

Make the chicken filling by adding the butter to a large saucepan over medium heat. Let it melt, then add the celery and onions and cook until soft.

Add the chicken broth, cream of chicken soup, salt and pepper. Stir until everything is well combined. Add the cooked chicken breast pieces and stir again. Cook for 5 minutes at a low simmer.

Transfer the filling mixture into 4 individual greased baking dishes or into a greased casserole dish. Top with the cornbread mixture and transfer to the oven.

Bake for 35-40 minutes for a large casserole dish or 25-30 minutes for individual dishes.

Nutrition: Calories: 454, Fat: 65 g, Carbs: 98 g, Protein: 88 g, Sodium: 387 mg

Sunday Chicken

Preparation Time: 10 minutes

Cooking Time: 10 minutes

Servings: 4

Ingredients:

Oil for frying

4 boneless, skinless chicken breasts

1 cups all-purpose flour

1 cup bread crumbs

2 teaspoons salt

2 teaspoons black pepper

1 cup buttermilk

½ cup water

Directions:

Add 3-4 inches of oil to a large pot or a deep fryer and preheat to 350°F.

Mix together the flour, breadcrumbs, salt and pepper in a shallow dish. To a separate shallow dish, add the buttermilk and water; stir.

Pound the chicken breasts to a consistent size. Dry them with a paper towel, then sprinkle with salt and pepper.

Dip the seasoned breasts in the flour mixture, then the buttermilk mixture, then back into the flour.

Add the breaded chicken to the hot oil and fry for about 8 minutes. Turn the chicken as necessary so that it cooks evenly on both sides.

Remove the chicken to either a wire rack or a plate lined with paper towels to drain.

Serve with mashed potatoes or whatever sides you love.

Nutrition: Calories:265, Fat: 47.9 g, Carbs: 65. 5 g, Protein: 37. 4 g, Sodium: 454 mg

Creamy Chicken and Rice

Preparation Time: 10 minutes

Cooking Time: 45 minutes

Servings: 4

Ingredients:

Salt and pepper to taste

2 cups cooked rice

1 diced onion

1 can cream of mushroom soup

1 packet chicken gravy

1½ pounds chicken breasts, cut into strips

Directions:

Preheat the oven to 350°F.

Cook the rice. When it is just about finished, toss in the diced onion so that it cooks too.

Prepare a baking dish by greasing or spraying with nonstick cooking spray.

Dump the rice into the prepared baking dish. Layer the chicken strips on top. Spread the undiluted cream of mushroom soup over the chicken.

In a small bowl, whisk together the chicken gravy with 1 cup of water, making sure to get all the lumps out. Pour this over the top of the casserole.

Cover with foil and transfer to the oven. Bake for 45 minutes or until the chicken is completely cooked.

Nutrition: Calories: 323, Fat: 56 g, Carbs: 32.5 g, Protein: 58.7 g, Sodium: 574 mg

Campfire Chicken

Preparation Time: 10 minutes

Cooking Time: 45 minutes

Servings: 4

Ingredients:

1 tablespoon paprika

2 teaspoons onion powder

2 teaspoons salt

1 teaspoon garlic powder

1 teaspoon dried rosemary

1 teaspoon black pepper

1 teaspoon dried oregano

1 whole chicken, quartered

2 carrots, cut into thirds

3 red skin potatoes, halved

1 ear of corn, quartered

1 tablespoon olive oil

1 tablespoon butter

5 sprigs fresh thyme

Directions:

Preheat the oven to 400°F.

In a small bowl, combine the paprika, onion powder, salt, garlic powder, rosemary, pepper and oregano.

Add the chicken quarters and 1 tablespoon of the spice mix to a large plastic freezer bag. Seal and refrigerate for at least 1 hour.

Add the corn, carrots and potatoes to a large bowl. Drizzle with the olive oil and remaining spice mix. Stir or toss to coat.

Preheat a large skillet over high heat. Add some oil, and when it is hot, add the chicken pieces and cook until golden brown.

Lay out 4 pieces of aluminum foil and add some carrots, potatoes, corn and a chicken quarter to each. Top with some butter and thyme.

Fold the foil in and make pouches by sealing the edges tightly.

Bake for 45 minutes.

Nutrition: Calories: 234, Fat: 54. 4 g, Carbs: 67. 9 g, Protein: 76. 5, Sodium: 652 mg

Chicken and Dumplings

Preparation Time: 30 minutes

Cooking Time: 20 minutes

Servings: 4

Ingredients:

2 cups flour

½ teaspoon baking powder 1 pinch salt

2 tablespoons butter   1 scant cup buttermilk

2 quarts chicken broth

3 cups cooked chicken

Directions:

Make the dumplings by combining the flour, baking powder and salt in a large bowl. Using a pastry cutter or two knives, cut the butter into the flour mixture. Stir in the milk a little at a time until it forms a dough ball.

Cover your countertop with enough flour that the dough will not stick when you roll it out. Roll out the dough relatively thin, then cut into squares to form dumplings.

Flour a plate and transfer the dough from the counter to the plate.

Bring the chicken broth to a boil in a large saucepan, then drop the dumplings in one by one, stirring continually. The excess flour will thicken the broth. Cook for about 20 minutes or until the dumplings are no longer doughy.

Add the chicken, stir to combine, and serve.

Nutrition: Calories: 323, Fat: 78 g, Carbs: 87 g, Protein: 69 g, Sodium: 769 mg

Chicken Pot Pie

Preparation Time: 30 minutes

Cooking Time: 30 minutes

Servings: 6 to 8

Ingredients:

½ cup butter

1 medium onion, diced

1 (14.5-ounce) can chicken broth

1 cup half and half milk

½ cup all-purpose flour

1 carrot, diced

1 celery stalk, diced

3 medium potatoes, peeled and diced

3 cups cooked chicken, diced

½ cup frozen peas

1 teaspoon chicken seasoning

½ teaspoon salt

½ teaspoon ground pepper

1 single refrigerated pie crust

1 egg

Water

Directions:

Preheat the oven to 375°F.

In a large skillet, heat the butter over medium heat, add the leeks and sauté for 3 minutes.

Sprinkle flour over the mixture, and continue to stir constantly for 3 minutes.

Whisking constantly, blend in the chicken broth and milk. Bring the mixture to a boil. Reduce heat to medium-low.

Add the carrots, celery, potatoes, salt, pepper, and stir to combine. Cook for 10-15 minutes or until veggies are cooked through but still crisp. Add chicken and peas. Stir to combine.

Transfer chicken filling to a deep 9-inch pie dish.

Fit the pie crust sheet on top and press the edges around the dish to seal the crust. Trim the excess if needed.

In a separate bowl, whisk an egg with 1 tablespoon of water, and brush the mixture over the top of the pie. With a knife, cut a few slits to let steam escape.

Bake the pie in the oven on the middle oven rack 20 to 30 minutes until the crust becomes golden brown.

Let the pie rest for about 15 minutes before serving.

Nutrition: Calories: 125, Fat: 43 g, Carbs: 76 g, Protein: 65 g, Sodium: 545 mg

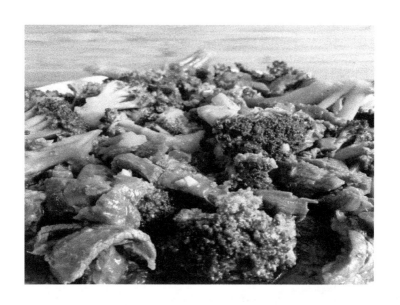

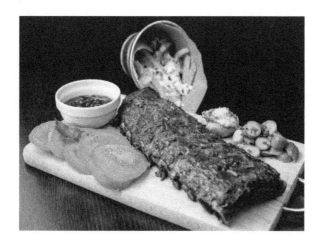

Compilation of Famous Main Dishes II

P.F. Chang's Mongolian Beef

Preparation Time: 10 minutes

Cooking Time: 20 minutes

Servings: 2

Ingredients:

1 pound flank steak

¼ cup cornstarch

2 teaspoons

½ teaspoon ginger, finely chopped

1 tablespoon ginger, diced

½ soy sauce

½ cup water

½ cup brown sugar

1 cup vegetable oil, divided

6 green onions, cut diagonally into 2-inch pieces

Directions:

Cut steak against the grain into small pieces, about ¼ inch. Transfer steak into a bowl with cornstarch and flip until fully coated on all sides. Set aside.

In a skillet, heat 1 tablespoon of the oil on medium heat. Stir in ginger and garlic. Cook for about 1 minute or until aromatic. Mix in soy sauce, water, and brown sugar. Keep stirring until sugar is melted. Bring to a boil on medium heat. Simmer for about 2 minutes or until sauce is thick.

Heat remaining vegetable oil in a separate saucepan on medium heat until oil reaches 350⁰F. Deep-fry steak in batches for 2 minutes or until brown. Transfer onto a plate lined with paper towels.

Discard the oil, then add sauce and stir in meat with sauce in saucepan for about 2 minutes on medium heat. Mix in green onions and cook for an additional 1-2 minute. Place meat and onions on a plate.

Serve hot.

Nutrition: Calories: 847, Fat: 24 g, Carbs: 103 g, Protein: 57 g, Sodium: 4176 mg

Panda Express' Beijing Beef

Preparation Time: 30 minutes

Cooking Time: 15 minutes

Servings: 4

Ingredients:

1 egg

¼ teaspoon salt

6 tablespoons water

9 tablespoons cornstarch

1 pound flank steak

4 tablespoons sugar

3 tablespoons ketchup

2 tablespoons vinegar

¼ teaspoon chili pepper, crushed

1 cup vegetable oil

1 teaspoon garlic, finely chopped

1 red bell pepper, chopped

1 green bell pepper, chopped

1 white onion, chopped

Directions:

To make the marinade, add egg, salt, 2 tablespoons water, and 1 tablespoon cornstarch in a bowl. Mix well.

Slice steak against the grain into small strips. Transfer into a Ziploc bag and pour marinade inside. Seal tightly. Shake bag gently to make sure the meat is well-coated. Set aside for at least 15 minutes.

To make the sauce, combine sugar, ketchup, vinegar, chili pepper, remaining 4 tablespoons water, and 2 teaspoons cornstarch in a bowl. Mix well. Cover and keep refrigerated.

Heat oil in a saucepan. Ready a bowl with 6 tablespoons cornstarch. Place beef in bowl and toss until fully coated. Shake off excess cornstarch and cook beef in hot oil until golden brown. Transfer onto a plate lined with paper towels.

Remove excess oil from saucepan. Toss in garlic, bell peppers, and onions and cook for about 2 minutes, stirring continuously. Transfer vegetables onto a plate.

In the same saucepan, add sauce and bring to a boil. Reduce heat to low and let simmer for 10 minutes.

Serve beef and vegetables with sauce poured on top.

Nutrition: Calories: 352, Fat: 11 g, Carbs: 36 g, Protein: 27 g, Sodium: 355 mg

Chili from Steak n' Shake

Preparation Time: 20 minutes

Cooking Time: 6 minutes

Servings: 6

Ingredients:

1 tablespoon olive oil

2 pounds ground beef

½ teaspoon salt

2 tablespoons onion powder

1 tablespoon chili powder

2 teaspoons ground cumin

½ teaspoon ground black pepper

2 teaspoons cocoa powder

6 ounces canned tomato paste

13½ ounces canned tomato sauce

1 cup Pepsi

27 ounces canned kidney beans, rinsed and drained

Shredded cheese, sliced green onions for toppings, if desired

Directions:

Heat oil in a pan. Add beef and cook until brown, drain, then remove from heat.

In a bowl, add cooked meat, salt, onion powder, chili powder, cumin, pepper, cocoa powder, tomato paste, tomato sauce, and Pepsi. Mix until combined.

Pour mixture into a blender and puree until well blended.

Add mixture into slow cooker. Pour in beans. Cover and set slow cooker to low setting and cook for 6 hours.

Serve with shredded cheese and green onions, if desired, on top.

Nutrition: Calories: 653, Fat: 41 g, Saturated fat: 17 g, Carbs: 38 g, Sugar: 12 g, Fibers: 11 g, Protein: 35 g, Sodium: 1308 mg

Cracker Barrel's Meatloaf

Preparation Time: 10 minutes

Cooking Time: 1 hour and 10 minutes

Servings: 4

Ingredients:

1 pound ground beef

1 onion, chopped

1 green pepper, chopped

1 can chopped tomatoes

1 egg

½ cup frozen biscuits, shredded

1 teaspoon salt

¼ cup ketchup (optional)

Non-stick cooking spray

Directions:

Preheat oven to 350°F.

In a bowl, add beef, onion, green pepper, tomatoes, egg, biscuits, and salt. Mix well.

Using a non-stick cooking spray, coat bread pan. Then, pour meatloaf mixture into pan. Make sure the mixture is even and flat in the pan.

Place in oven and bake for about 1 hour and 5 minutes or until cooked through. Remove from oven and allow to cool for about 10 minutes.

Drain excess juice, then invert cooked meatloaf onto a serving plate. Drizzle ketchup on top, if desired. Serve.

Nutrition: Calories: 485, Fat: 32 g, Saturated Fat: 13 g, Carbs: 27 g, Sugar: 3 g, Fibers: 1 g, Protein: 23 g, Sodium: 1273 mg

DIY Sizzling Steak, Cheese, and Mushrooms Skillet from Applebee's

Preparation Time: 15 minutes

Cooking Time: 1 hour and 35 minutes

Servings: 4

Ingredients:

1 head garlic, cut crosswise

2 tablespoons olive oil, divided

Salt and pepper, to taste

2 pounds Yukon Gold potatoes, chopped into 1-inch pieces

Water, for boiling

2 tablespoons butter

1 large yellow onion

8 ounces cremini mushrooms

Salt and pepper to taste

½ cup milk

¼ cup cream

3 tablespoons butter

2½ pounds 1-inch thick sirloin steak, cut into 4 large pieces

8 slices mozzarella cheese

Directions:

Preheat oven to 300°F.

Position garlic on foil. Pour 1 tablespoon olive oil to the inner sides where the garlic was cut, then wrap foil around garlic.

Place in oven and bake for 30 minutes. Remove from oven, and squeeze out garlic from head. Transfer to a bowl or mortar. Add salt and pepper, then mash together. Set aside.

In a pot, add potatoes. Pour enough water on top to cover potatoes. Bring to a boil. Once boiling, reduce heat to medium. Simmer for about 20 to 25 minutes or until potatoes become tender.

Melt butter on a non-stick pan over medium-low heat. Add onions and sauté for about 15 minutes until a bit tender. Toss in mushrooms and sauté, adjusting heat to medium. Season with salt and pepper. Cook for 10 minutes more. Set aside and keep warm.

Drain potatoes, then mash using an electric mixer on low speed. While mashing, gradually pour in milk, cream, butter, and mashed garlic with olive oil. Keep blending until everything is cream-like and smooth. Remove from mixer and place a cover on top of bowl. Set aside and keep warm.

Evenly coat steak pieces with remaining 1 tablespoon olive oil on all sides. Heat grill, then place meat on grill. Cook for 4 minutes. Flip and add mozzarella slices on top. Cook for another 4 minutes for medium rare. Add additional minutes for increased doneness.

Transfer steaks to serving plates then top with onion/mushroom mixture. Place mashed potatoes on the side. Serve.

Nutrition: Calories: 1159, Fat: 60 g, Saturated Fat: 29 g, Carbs: 47 g, Sugar: 4 g, Fibers: 6 g, Protein: 107 g, Sodium: 1495 mg

Panda Express' Copycat Beef and Broccoli

Preparation Time: 30 minutes

Cooking Time: 15 minutes

Servings: 4

Ingredients:

2 tablespoons cornstarch, divided

3 tablespoons Chinese rice wine, divided

1 pound flank steak, cut thinly against the grain

1 pound broccoli florets, chopped into small pieces

2 tablespoons oyster sauce   2 tablespoons water

1 tablespoon brown sugar   1 tablespoon soy sauce

1 tablespoon cornstarch

2 tablespoons canola oil

¼ teaspoon sesame oil

1 teaspoon ginger, finely chopped

2 cloves garlic, finely chopped

2 teaspoons sesame seeds

Directions:

In a large Ziploc bag, add 1 tablespoon cornstarch and 2 tablespoons Chinese rice wine. Place beef inside and seal tightly. Massage bag to fully coat beef. Set aside to marinate for at least 20 minutes.

Rinse broccoli and place in a nonreactive bowl. Place a wet paper towel on top, then microwave for 2 minutes. Set aside.

Stir oyster sauce, water, 1 tablespoon Chinese rice wine, brown sugar, soy sauce, and remaining cornstarch in a bowl until well mixed. Set aside.

Heat wok over high heat. You want the wok to be very hot. Then, heat canola and sesame oil in wok and wait to become hot.

Working in batches, add steak and cook over high heat for 1 minute. Flip, and cook other side for another 1 minute. Transfer to a plate.

To the same wok, add garlic and ginger. Sauté for about 10 to 15 seconds then return beef to wok. Toss in heated broccoli. Slightly stir prepared sauce to make sure cornstarch is not settled on the bottom, then add to wok. Toss everything in sauce to combine. Continue cooking until sauce becomes thick. Garnish with sesame seeds. Serve.

Nutrition: Calories: 324, Fat: 17 g, Saturated Fat: 4g, Carbs: 13 g, Sugar: 6g, Fibers: 3 g, Protein: 28 g, Sodium: 464 mg

Jack Daniel's Ribs from TGI Fridays

Preparation Time: 15 minutes

Cooking Time: 5 minutes

Servings: 4

Ingredients:

1 head garlic

1 tablespoon olive oil 1½ teaspoons paprika

½ teaspoon salt ¼ teaspoon dried thyme

½ teaspoon ground black pepper

½ teaspoon garlic powder

½ teaspoon onion powder

¼ teaspoon celery salt

¼ teaspoon ground cayenne pepper

2 racks baby back ribs

½ cup water

1 cup pineapple juice

¼ cup teriyaki sauce

1 tablespoon soy sauce

1⅓ cups dark brown sugar

3 tablespoons lemon juice

¼ cup white onion, finely chopped

2 tablespoons Jack Daniel's whiskey

1 heaping tablespoon pineapple, crushed

¼ teaspoon cayenne pepper

Directions:

Preheat oven to 300°F.

Take garlic and chop off about ½ inches from the head. Take out paper-like outer layers then place in a small oven-safe bowl or ramekin. Pour olive oil on top and wrap in aluminum foil. Place in oven and bake for 1 hour. When ready, remove from oven and allow to cool. Squeeze out about garlic from roasted garlic head. Add roasted garlic in an airtight container and plce in refrigerator

While the garlic is baking, prepare the spice rub by combining paprika, salt, thyme, pepper, garlic powder, onion powder, celery salt, and ground cayenne pepper in a bowl. Mix well. Evenly coat ribs with spice rub. Arrange ribs onto a baking sheet. Bake in oven for about 2½ hours.

Prepare the barbecue sauce by mixing water, pineapple juice, teriyaki sauce, soy sauce, and dark brown sugar in a pan. Bring to a boil while stirring from time to time. Once boiling, lower heat until mixture is just simmering.

Add to pan 2 teaspoons of the roasted garlic, lemon juice, onion, whiskey, crushed pineapple, and cayenne pepper. Stir to combine well. Simmer for about 30 to 40 minutes until liquid is reduced by half.

If desired, you can finish the ribs on the barbecue to have grilling marks and crisper ribs. Preheat grill to medium-high heat. Then, place ribs onto grill and cook for about 2 to 4 minutes. Turn ribs over and grill for another 2 to 4 minutes.

Transfer onto a serving plate. Spoon sauce over ribs. Serve.

Nutrition: Calories: 779, Fat: 38 g, Saturated Fat: 13 g, Carbs: 80 g, Sugar: 77 g, Fibers: 1 g, Protein: 29 g, Sodium: 865 mg

Smokehouse Pork Belly Sandwich from Arby's

Preparation Time: 15 minutes

Cooking Time: 2 hours and 30 minutes

Servings: 6

Ingredients:

2 pounds center cut pork belly

Salt and pepper, to taste

1-2 tablespoons barbecue spice rub

6 star cross buns

Cooking spray

½ pound smoked cheddar cheese

½ cup mayonnaise

½ cup any smoky barbecue sauce

6 ounces onion strings

Directions:

Sprinkle salt and pepper onto pork belly then coat with barbecue rub.

Set smoker to 300°F with hickory wood on coals. Put pork belly in smoker with fat side facing down.

Smoke for about 2½ hours until well browned and a bit charred. Pork is ready once its internal temperature is about 185 to 195°F.

Spray cooking spray onto the inner sides of buns then toast until golden brown.

Assemble sandwich by layering mayo, cooked pork belly, barbecue sauce, cheese, and onion strings on the bottom bun. Top with second bun. Repeat for remaining sandwiches.

Serve.

Nutrition: Calories: 1351, Fat: 117 g, Saturated Fat: 41 g, Carbs: 45 g, Sugar: 13 g, Fibers: 2 g, Protein: 29 g, Sodium: 1023 mg

Red Beans and Rice from Popeye's

Preparation Time: 20 minutes

Cooking Time: 40 minutes

Servings: 10

Ingredients:

3 14-ounce cans red beans

¾ pounds smoked ham hock

1¼ cups water

½ teaspoon onion powder

½ teaspoon garlic salt

¼ teaspoon red pepper flakes

½ teaspoon salt

3 tablespoons lard

Steamed long-grain rice

Directions:

Add 2 canned red beans, ham hock, and water to pot. Cook on medium heat and let simmer for about 1 hour.

Remove from heat and wait until meat is cool enough to handle. Then, remove meat from bone.

In a food processor, add meat, cooked red beans and water mixture, onion powder, garlic salt, red pepper, salt, and lard. Pulse for 4 seconds. You want the beans to be cut and the liquid thickened. Drain remaining 1 can red beans and add to food processor. Pulse for only 1 or 2 seconds.

Remove ingredients from food processor and transfer to the pot from earlier. Cook on low heat, stirring frequently until mixture is heated through.

Serve over steamed rice.

Nutrition: Calories: 445, Fat: 12 g, Saturated Fat: 4g, Carbs: 67 g, Sugar: 1 g, Fibers: 9 g, Protein: 17 g, Sodium: 670 mg

Café Rio's Sweet Pork Barbacoa Salad

Preparation Time: 10 minutes

Cooking Time: 8 minutes

Servings: 8

Ingredients:

3 pounds pork loin

Garlic salt, to taste

1 can root beer

¼ cup water

¾ cup brown sugar

1 10-ounce can red enchilada sauce

1 4-ounce can green chilies

½ teaspoon chili powder

8 large burrito size tortillas

1½ serving Cilantro Lime Rice

1 can black beans, drained and heated

2 heads Romaine lettuce, shredded

1½ cups tortilla strips

1 cup Queso Fresco cheese

2 limes, cut in wedges

¼ cup cilantro

Dressing:

½ packet Hidden Valley Ranch Dressing Mix

1 cup mayonnaise

½ cup milk

½ cup cilantro leaves

¼ cup salsa verde

½ jalapeno pepper, deseeded

1 plump clove garlic

2 tablespoons fresh lime juice

Directions:

Sprinkle garlic salt on pork. Put in slow cooker with the fat side facing down. Add ¼ cup root beer and water. Cover and cook on low setting for 6 hours.

To prepare sauce add the rest of the root beer, brown sugar, enchilada sauce, green chilies, and chili powder in a blender. Blend until smooth.

Remove meat from slow cooker then transfer onto cutting board. Shred, discarding juices and fat. Return shredded pork to slow cooker with sauce. Cook on low setting for another 2 hours. When there is only about 15 to 20 minutes left to cook, remove lid to thicken sauce.

To prepare dressing mix all dressing ingredients in a blender. Puree until smooth. Then, transfer to refrigerator and allow to chill for at least 1 hour.

To assemble salad, layer tortilla, rice, beans, pork, lettuce, tortilla strips, cheese, and dressing in a bowl. Serve with a lime wedge and cilantro leaves.

Nutrition: Calories: 756, Fat: 28 g, Saturated Fat: 7 g, Carbs: 91 g, Sugar: 31 g, Fibers: 7 g, Protein: 38 g, Sodium: 1389 mg

Edo Japan's Sukiyaki Beef

Preparation Time: 15 minutes

Cooking Time: 5 to 6 minutes

Marinating Time: 20 minutes

Servings: 2 to 4

Ingredients:

10 ounces sirloin steak, thinly sliced

½ carrot, thinly sliced

½ onion, sliced

1 green pepper, sliced

½ yellow bell pepper, sliced

½ cup sukiyaki sauce, divided

1 tablespoon oil

1 teaspoon chopped garlic

2 tablespoons ginger, finely chopped

2 teaspoons soy sauce

1 teaspoon sugar

1 tablespoon oyster sauce

Directions:

Pour half of the sukiyaki sauce into a medium bowl and add the sliced beef. Let the beef marinate for 20 minutes.

Heat the oil in a large skillet. Add the garlic and cook for about 30 seconds.

Add the beef, with the sauce. Cook over medium-high heat until the beef is cooked through.

Add the ginger, carrots, peppers and onions and cook until the veggies have begun to soften.

Add the rest of the sukiyaki sauce along with the oyster sauce, soy sauce and sugar. Cook and stir for about 2 more minutes.

Serve over rice.

Nutrition: Calories: 152, Fat:24 g, Carbs: 20 g, Protein: 5.6 g, Sodium: 627 mg

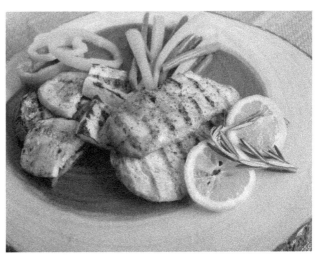

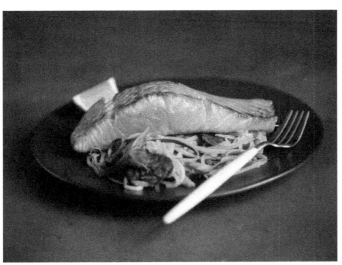

Compilation of Main Dishes III

Chicken Fried Chicken

Preparation Time: 15 minutes

Cooking Time: 30 minutes

Servings: 4

Ingredients:

Chicken

½ cup all-purpose flour

1 teaspoon poultry seasoning

½ teaspoon salt

½ teaspoon pepper

1 egg, slightly beaten

1 tablespoon water

4 boneless skinless chicken breasts, pounded to ½-inch thickness

1 cup vegetable oil

Gravy

2 tablespoons all-purpose flour

¼ teaspoon salt

¼ teaspoon pepper

1¼ cups milk

Directions:

Preheat the oven to 200°F.

In a shallow dish, combine the flour, poultry seasoning, salt and pepper.

In another shallow dish, mix together the beaten egg and water.

First dip both sides of the chicken breasts in the flour mixture, then dip them in the egg mixture, and then back into the flour mixture.

Heat the vegetable oil over medium-high heat in a large deep skillet. A cast iron is good choice if you have one. Add the chicken and cook for about 15 minutes, or until fully cooked, turning over about halfway through.

Transfer the chicken to a cookie sheet and place in the oven to maintain temperature.

Remove all but 2 tablespoons of oil from the skillet you cooked the chicken in.

Prepare the gravy by whisking the dry gravy ingredients together in a bowl. Then whisk them into the oil in the skillet, stirring thoroughly to remove lumps. When the flour begins to brown, slowly whisk in the milk. Continue cooking and whisking for about 2 minutes or until the mixture thickens.

Top chicken with some of the gravy.

Nutrition: Calories: 234, Fat: 24 g, Carbs: 54 g, Protein: 61 g, Sodium: 1286 mg

Broccoli Cheddar Chicken

Preparation Time: 10 minutes

Cooking Time: 45 minutes

Servings: 4

Ingredients:

4 skinless chicken breasts

1 cup milk

1 cup Ritz-style crackers, crushed

1 (10.5-ounce) can condensed cheddar cheese soup

½ pound frozen broccoli

6 ounces cheddar cheese, shredded

½ teaspoon salt

½ teaspoon pepper

Directions:

Preheat the oven to 350°F.

Whisk the milk and cheddar cheese soup together in a mixing bowl.

Prepare a baking dish by greasing the sides, then lay the chicken in the bottom and season with the salt and pepper.

Pour the soup mixture over the chicken, then top with the crackers, broccoli and shredded cheese.

Bake for about 45 minutes or until bubbly.

Nutrition: Calories: 343, Fat: 43 g, Carbs: 54 g, Protein: 16 g, Sodium: 565 mg

Cajun Jambalaya Pasta

Preparation Time: 10 minutes

Cooking Time: 50 minutes

Servings: 6

Ingredients:

¼ cup unsalted butter

¼ cup extra-virgin olive oil

1 pound andouille sausage or smoked sausage, sliced

1 pound boneless skinless chicken breast, cubed

1 bell pepper, diced

1 white onion, diced

3 stalks celery, diced

4 cloves garlic, minced

1 pound jumbo shrimp, peeled and deveined

2 cups red salsa

1 (6 -ounce) can hot tomato sauce

1 quart low-sodium chicken broth

1 bay leaf

¼ cup Italian parsley, chopped

½ bunch green onions

1 pound linguine pasta, cooked according to the package directions

Spice Blend

1 tablespoon creole seasoning

1 tablespoon garlic powder

1 tablespoon onion powder

2 teaspoons black pepper

1 teaspoon paprika

Pinch cayenne pepper

Garlic bread, for serving

Directions:

In a small dish, mix together all the spices for the spice blend.

Season the chicken chunks with 1 tablespoon of the spice blend. Mix until the chicken is well coated, and set it aside.

In a large saucepan, melt the butter and heat olive oil over medium heat.

When it is hot, add the sausage slices and cook for 5 minutes. Add the chicken and cook for about 10 minutes.

Next, add the bell pepper, onion, and celery. Mix in half of the remaining spice blend. Cook for approximately 10 minutes, then add the garlic and cook 1 more minute.

With 1 tablespoon of seasoning blend, season the shrimp and set it aside. Then add the rest of the spices to the saucepan and stir to combine.

Add the salsa, tomato sauce, chicken broth, and the bay leaf. Mix together and bring it to a boil, stirring it together so that everything is well combined. Don't forget to scrape the bottom of the pan for brown bits.

Reduce the heat and let it simmer, covered, for about 30 minutes. Once the 30 minutes is up, discard the bay leaf. Add the shrimp, parsley, and green onions, and cook, still covered for about 10 minutes more.

Serve over pasta with a slice of toasted garlic bread.

Nutrition: Calories: 234, Fat: 53 g, Carbs: 65 g, Protein: 62 g, Sodium: 652 mg

Grilled Chicken Tenderloin

Preparation Time: 10 minutes

 Marinating Time: 1 hour

Cooking Time: 30 min

Servings: 4 to 5

Ingredients:

4-5 boneless and skinless chicken breasts, cut into strips, or 12 chicken tenderloins, tendons removed

1 cup Italian dressing

2 teaspoons lime juice

4 teaspoons honey

Directions:

Combine the dressing, lime juice and honey in a plastic bag. Seal and shake to combine.

Place the chicken in the bag. Seal and shake again, then transfer to the refrigerator for at least 1 hour. The longer it marinates, the more the flavors will infuse into the chicken.

When ready to prepare, transfer the chicken and the marinade to a large nonstick skillet.

Bring to a boil, then reduce the heat and allow simmering until the liquid has cooked down to a glaze.

Nutrition: Calories: 451, Fat: 43 g, Carbs: 61 g, Protein: 65.7 g, Sodium: 526 mg

Miso Glazed Salmon

Preparation Time: 10 minutes

Cooking Time: 10 minutes

Servings: 4

Ingredients:

½ cup brown sugar

3 tablespoons soy sauce

¼ cup hot water

3 tablespoons miso (soybean paste)

4 salmon fillets

1 tablespoon butter

2 tablespoons ginger paste

1 tablespoon garlic paste

½ cup sake

1 tablespoon heavy cream

½ cup butter, cut into 8 pieces

Juice of half of a lime

For serving:

Steamed snow peas, broccoli, and carrots

Steamed Jasmine Rice

Directions:

Preheat the broiler.

Mix together the brown sugar, soy sauce, hot water, and miso paste. Stir until well combined.

Lightly oil a baking dish and arrange the salmon fillets in it. Spoon some of the miso mixture over each fillet, leaving some for basting. Transfer the pan to the oven and broil for about 10 minutes. Baste every 3 minutes while broiling.

In the meantime, in a small saucepan, melt 1 tablespoon of butter over medium-high heat. Add the ginger and garlic paste, and cook for about 2 minutes.

Stir in the sake and bring the mixture to a boil. Let it cook for 3 more minutes, and add the heavy cream. Cook another 2 minutes, or until the sauce starts to reduce. Then whisk in the remaining butter one piece at a time and cook until the sauce thickens. Remove the saucepan from the heat and stir in the lime juice.

When the salmon is done, serve by pouring a little sauce over the rice and top with a salmon fillet with vegetables on the side.

Nutrition: Calories: 234, Fat: 34.9 g, Carbs: 43 g, Protein: 45 g, Sodium: 524 mg

Almond Crusted Salmon Salad

Preparation Time: 15 minutes

Cooking Time: 30 minutes

Servings: 4

Ingredients:

¼ cup olive oil

4 (4 -ounce) portions salmon

½ teaspoon kosher salt

⅛ teaspoon ground black pepper

2 tablespoons garlic aioli (bottled is fine)

½ cup chopped and ground almonds for crust

10 ounces kale, chopped

¼ cup lemon dressing of choice

2 avocados, peeled, pitted and cut into ½-inch pieces

2 cups cooked quinoa

1 cup brussels sprouts, sliced

2 ounces arugula

½ cup dried cranberries

1 cup balsamic vinaigrette

24 thin radish slices

Lemon zest

Directions:

In a large skillet, heat the olive oil over medium-high heat. Sprinkle the salmon with salt and pepper to season. When the skillet is hot, add the fish fillets and cook for about 3 minutes on each side, or until it flakes easily with a fork. Top the salmon with garlic aioli and sprinkle with nuts.

Meanwhile, combine all the salad ingredients, including the quinoa, in a bowl and toss with the dressing.

Serve the salad with a fish fillet on top of greens and sprinkle with radishes and lemon zest.

Nutrition: Calories: 243, Fat: 45 g, Carbs: 23 g, Protein: 52 g, Sodium: 1436 mg

Shrimp Scampi

Preparation Time: 10 minutes

Cooking Time: 30 minutes

Servings: 4

Ingredients:

1–2 pounds fresh shrimp, cleaned, deveined, and butterflied

1 cup milk

3 tablespoons olive oil

½ cup all-purpose flour

4 tablespoons Parmesan cheese, divided

¼ teaspoon salt

½ teaspoon fresh ground black pepper

¼ teaspoon cayenne pepper

6–8 whole garlic cloves

1 cup dry white wine

2 cups heavy cream

5–7 leaves fresh basil, cut into strips

1 diced tomato

2 tablespoons Parmesan cheese, finely grated

1 shallot, diced

1 pound angel hair pasta, cooked (hot)

Parsley, to garnish

Directions:

Put the shrimp in the milk and let it sit.

In a shallow bowl, combine the flour, 2 tablespoons of Parmesan, salt, pepper, and cayenne.

Pour the olive oil in a large skillet, making sure it's enough to cover the bottom. Heat over medium-high heat.

Take the shrimp from the milk and dredge in flour mixture. Transfer it to the skillet and cook about 2 minutes on each side. After the shrimp cooks, transfer it to a plate covered with a paper towel to drain.

Reduce the heat to medium-low and cook the garlic in the leftover oil. (Don't worry about any bits left from the shrimp because these will add flavor and help to thicken the sauce.)

After the garlic cooks for a couple of minutes, add the wine. Increase the heat and bring the mixture to a boil, then reduce the heat and simmer to reduce liquid to about half of the original volume.

Add the cream and simmer for about 10 more minutes, then add the basil, tomato, cheese, and shallots. Stir to combine.

Add the shrimp to the skillet and remove it from the heat.

Arrange the pasta on serving plates, topped with shrimp and covered with sauce. Garnish with parsley.

Nutrition: Calories: 454, Fat: 54 g, Carbs: 152 g, Protein: 41 g, Sodium: 1614 mg

Copycat Wendy's Beef Chili

Preparation Time: 15 minutes

Cooking Time: 1 hour and 20 minutes

Servings: 10

Ingredients:

2 tablespoons olive oil

2 pounds ground beef

2 stalks celery, diced

1 onion, diced

1 green bell pepper, diced

3 14-ounce cans stewed tomatoes

1 10-ounce can diced tomatoes with green chiles (such as Ro*Tel)

1 14-ounce can tomato sauce

1 cup water

2 1¼- ounce packages chili seasoning

1 14-ounce can kidney beans, not drained

1 14-ounce can pinto beans, not drained

Salt and ground black pepper to taste

1 tablespoon white vinegar

Directions:

In a pot, cook oil on medium-high heat. Add beef and cook for 8-10 minutes or until beef is brown, crumbly, and cooked through.

Toss in celery, onion, and bell pepper into pot. Sauté for 5 minutes or until fragrant. Add stewed and diced tomatoes, green chilies, tomato sauce, and water. Stir until there are no more big chunks from the stewed tomatoes, then mix in chili seasoning.

Add kidney and pinto beans into pot. Sprinkle salt and pepper, to taste. Stir, and bring to a boil. Then reduce heat to a simmer. Simmer for about 1 hour on low heat. Stir in vinegar. Serve hot.

Nutrition: Calories: 326, Fat: 15 g, Carbs: 29 g, Protein: 23 g, Sodium: 1521 mg

The Mexican Pizza from Taco Bell

Preparation Time: 30 minutes

Cooking Time: 12 minutes

Servings: 4

Ingredients:

½ pound ground beef

½ teaspoon salt

¼ teaspoon onion, finely chopped

¼ teaspoon paprika

1½ teaspoon chili powder

2 tablespoons water

1 cup vegetable oil

8 6-inch flour tortillas

1 16-ounce can refried beans

⅔ cup picante sauce

⅓ cup tomato, finely chopped

1 cup cheddar cheese, grated

1 cup Colby jack cheese, grated

¼ cup green onion, diced

¼ cup black olives, chopped

Directions:

Preheat oven to 400°F.

In a skillet, sauté beef on medium heat. Once brown, drain. Then stir in salt, onions, paprika, chili powder, and water. While continuously stirring, cook for an additional 10 minutes.

In a separate skillet add oil and heat over medium-high. Cook tortilla for about 30 seconds on both sides or until golden brown. Use a fork to pierce any bubbles forming on the tortillas. Transfer onto a plate lined with paper towels.

Microwave refried beans on high for about 30 seconds or until warm.

To build each pizza, coat ⅓ cup beans on tortilla followed by ⅓ cup cooked beef. Top with a second tortilla. Cover with 2 tablespoons picante sauce, then equal amounts of tomatoes, cheeses, green onions, and olives. This makes a total of 4 pizzas.

Place prepared pizzas on baking sheet. Bake in oven until cheese is fully melted, about 8 to 12 minutes.

Serve.

Nutrition: Calories: 1218, Fat: 90 g, Carbs: 66 g, Protein: 39 g, Sodium: 2038 mg

Copycat Swedish Meatballs from Ikea

Preparation Time: 30 minutes

Cooking Time: 30 minutes

Servings: 2

Ingredients:

3 tablespoons butter, divided

1¼ tablespoon onion, minced

1 boiled potato, cold

¼ ground beef

¼ ground pork

1 egg

¼ cup milk

¼ cup water

⅛ cup breadcrumbs

Salt, to taste

White pepper, to taste

Sauce

1 tablespoon all-purpose flour

1 tablespoon butter

½ cup beef stock

¼ cup cream

For serving

Boiled potatoes

Lingonberry jam

Directions:

To make the meatballs, melt 2 tablespoons of the butter in a pan over medium-high heat. Add onion and cook until transparent, about 1-2 minutes.

In a bowl, mash a potato. Then, combine with cooked onion, beef, pork, egg, milk, water, and breadcrumbs. Season salt and white pepper, to taste.

Flour cutting board and form meat into round 1-inch balls.

In previous pan, melt remaining butter and cook on low heat until meatballs are cooked through, about 4-6 minutes, stirring a few times. Don't overcrowd the pan, work in batch if needed.

Transfer to a plate and cover with foil to keep warm.

To make the sauce, heat butter in a saucepan over medium heat. Stir in flour and cook until golden brown. Pour in stock and cream, and whisk until smooth. Flavor with salt and pepper, to taste.

Pour sauce onto meatballs and serve with boiled potatoes and lingonberry jam.

Nutrition: Calories: 1172, Fat: 87 g, Carbs: 45 g, Protein: 52 g, Sodium: 520 mg

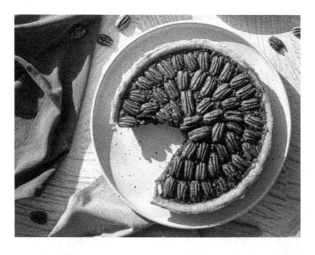

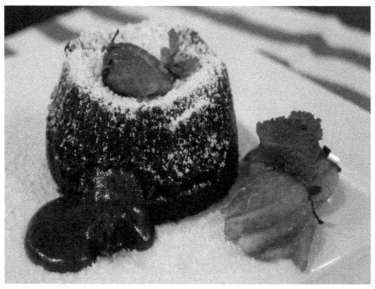

Desserts

Cinnamon Apple Turnover

Preparation Time: 10 minutes

Cooking Time: 25 minutes

Servings: 4 to 6

Ingredients:

1 large Granny Smith apple, peeled, cored, and diced

$\frac{1}{2}$ teaspoon cornstarch

$\frac{1}{4}$ teaspoon cinnamon

Dash ground nutmeg

$\frac{1}{4}$ cup brown sugar

$\frac{1}{4}$ cup applesauce

$\frac{1}{4}$ teaspoon vanilla extract

1 tablespoon butter, melted

1 sheet of puff pastry, thawed

Whipped cream or vanilla ice cream, to serve

Directions:

Preheat the oven to 400°F.

Prepare a baking sheet by spraying it with non-stick cooking spray or using a bit of oil on a paper towel.

In a mixing bowl, mix together the apples, cornstarch, cinnamon, nutmeg, and brown sugar. Stir to make sure the apples are well covered with the spices. Then stir in the applesauce and the vanilla.

Lay out your puff pastry and cut it into squares. You should be able to make 4 or 6 depending on how big you want your turnovers to be and how big your pastry is.

Place some of the apple mixture in the center of each square and fold the corners of the pastry up to make a pocket. Pinch the edges together to seal. Then brush a bit of the melted butter over the top to give the turnovers that nice brown color.

Place the filled pastry onto the prepared baking pan and transfer to the preheated oven. Bake 20–25 minutes, or until they become a golden brown in color.

Serve with whipped cream or vanilla ice cream.

Nutrition: Calories: 332, Fat: 24 g, Carbs: 65 g, Protein: 76 g, Sodium: 767 mg

Cherry Chocolate Cobbler

Preparation Time: 10 minutes

Cooking Time: 45 minutes

Servings: 8

Ingredients:

1½ cups all-purpose flour

½ cup sugar

2 teaspoons baking powder

½ teaspoon salt

¼ cup butter

6 ounces semisweet chocolate morsels

¼ cup milk

1 egg, beaten

21 ounces cherry pie filling

½ cup finely chopped nuts

Directions:

Preheat the oven to 350°F.

Combine the flour, sugar, baking powder, salt and butter in a large mixing bowl. Use a pastry blender to cut the mixture until there are lumps the size of small peas.

Melt the chocolate morsels. Let cool for approximately 5 minutes, then add the milk and egg and mix well. Beat into the flour mixture, mixing completely.

Spread the pie filling in a 2-quart casserole dish. Randomly drop the chocolate batter over the filling, and then sprinkle with nuts.

Bake for 40–45 minutes.

Serve with a scoop of vanilla ice cream if desired.

Nutrition: Calories: 243, Fat: 41 g, Carbs: 75 g, Protein: 67 g, Sodium: 879 mg

Chocolate Pecan Pie

Preparation Time: 10 minutes

Cooking Time: 50 minutes

Servings: 8

Ingredients:

3 eggs

½ cup sugar

1 cup corn syrup

½ teaspoon salt

1 teaspoon vanilla extract

¼ cup melted butter

1 cup pecans

3 tablespoons semisweet chocolate chips

1 unbaked pie shell

Directions:

Preheat the oven to 350°F.

Beat together the eggs and sugar in a mixing bowl, then add the corn syrup, salt, vanilla and butter.

Put the chocolate chips and pecans inside the pie shell and pour the egg mixture over the top.

Bake for 50-60 minutes or until set.

Serve with vanilla ice cream.

Nutrition: Calories: 465, Fat: 76 g, Carbs: 37 g, Protein: 97 g, Sodium: 4461 mg

Pumpkin Custard with Gingersnaps

Preparation Time: 30 minutes

Cooking Time: 35 minutes

Servings: 8

Ingredients:

Custard

8 egg yolks

1¾ cups (1 15-ounce can) pure pumpkin puree

1¾ cups heavy whipping cream

½ cup sugar

1½ teaspoons pumpkin pie spice

1 teaspoon vanilla

Topping

1 cup crushed gingersnap cookies

1 tablespoon melted butter

Whipped Cream

1 cup heavy whipping cream

1 tablespoon superfine sugar (or regular sugar if you have no caster sugar)

½ teaspoon pumpkin pie spice

Garnish

8 whole gingersnap cookies

Directions:

Preheat the oven to 350°F.

Separate the yolks from 8 eggs and whisk them together in a large mixing bowl until they are well blended and creamy.

Add the pumpkin, sugar, vanilla, heavy cream and pumpkin pie spice and whisk to combine.

Cook the custard mixture in a double boiler, stirring until it has thickened enough that it coats a spoon.

Pour the mixture into individual custard cups or an 8×8-inch baking pan and bake for about 20 minutes if using individual cups or 30–35 minutes for the baking pan, until it is set, and a knife inserted comes out clean.

While the custard is baking, make the topping by combining the crushed gingersnaps and melted butter. After the custard has been in the oven for 15 minutes, sprinkle the gingersnap mixture over the top.

When the custard has passed the clean knife test, remove from the oven and let cool to room temperature.

Whisk the heavy cream and pumpkin pie spice together with the caster sugar and beat just until it thickens.

Serve the custard with the whipped cream and garnish each serving with a gingersnap.

Nutrition: Calories: 255, Fat: 35 g, Carbs: 25 g, Protein: 76 g, Sodium: 877 mg

Baked Apple Dumplings

Preparation Time: 20 minutes

Cooking Time: 40 minutes

Servings: 2 to 4

Ingredients:

1 (17½ ounce) package frozen puff pastry, thawed

1 cup sugar

6 tablespoons dry breadcrumbs

2 teaspoons ground cinnamon

1 pinch ground nutmeg

1 egg, beaten

4 Granny Smith apples, peeled, cored and halved

Vanilla ice cream for serving

Icing

1 cup confectioners' sugar

1 teaspoon vanilla extract

3 tablespoons milk

Pecan Streusel

⅔ cup chopped toasted pecans

⅔ cup packed brown sugar

⅔ cup all-purpose flour

5 tablespoons melted butter

Directions:

Preheat the oven to 425°F.

When the puff pastry has completely thawed, roll out each sheet to measure 12 inches by 12 inches. Cut the sheets into quarters.

Combine the sugar, breadcrumbs, cinnamon and nutmeg together in a small bowl.

Brush one of the pastry squares with some of the beaten egg. Add about 1 tablespoon of the breadcrumb mixture on top, then add half an apple, core side down, over the crumbs. Add another tablespoon of the breadcrumb mixture.

Seal the dumpling by pulling up the corners and pinching the pastry together until the seams are totally sealed. Repeat this process with the remaining squares.

Assemble the ingredients for the pecan streusel in a small bowl.

Grease a baking sheet, or line it with parchment paper. Place the dumplings on the sheet and brush them with a bit more of the beaten egg. Top with the pecan streusel.

Bake for 15 minutes, then reduce heat to 350°F and bake for 25 minutes more or until lightly browned.

Make the icing by combining the confectioners' sugar, vanilla and milk until you reach the proper consistency.

When the dumplings are done, let them cool to room temperature and drizzle them with icing before serving.

Nutrition: Calories:145, Fat: 57 g, Carbs: 87 g, Protein: 66.9 g, Sodium: 529 mg

Peach Cobbler

Preparation Time: 10 minutes

Cooking Time: 45 minutes

Servings: 4

Ingredients:

1¼ cups Bisquick

1 cup milk

½ cup melted butter

¼ teaspoon nutmeg

½ teaspoon cinnamon

Vanilla ice cream, for serving

Filling

1 (30-ounce) can peaches in syrup, drained

¼ cup sugar

Topping

½ cup brown sugar

¼ cup almond slices

½ teaspoon cinnamon

1 tablespoon melted butter

Directions:

Preheat the oven to 375°F.

Grease the bottom and sides of an 8×8-inch pan.

Whisk together the Bisquick, milk, butter, nutmeg and cinnamon in a large mixing bowl. When thoroughly combined, pour into the greased baking pan.

Mix together the peaches and sugar in another mixing bowl. Put the filling on top of the batter in the pan. Bake for about 45 minutes.

In another bowl, mix together the brown sugar, almonds, cinnamon, and melted butter. After the cobbler has cooked for 45 minutes, cover evenly with the topping and bake for an additional 10 minutes.

Serve with a scoop of vanilla ice cream.

Nutrition: Calories: 168, Fat: 76 g, Carbs: 15 g, Protein: 78.9 g, Sodium: 436 mg

Royal Dansk Butter Cookies

Preparation Time: 15 minutes

Cooking Time: 25 minutes

Servings: 10

Ingredients:

120g cake flour, sifted

½ teaspoon vanilla extract

25g powdered sugar

120g softened butter, at room temperature

A pinch of sea salt, approximately ¼ teaspoon

Directions:

Using a hand mixer; beat the butter with sugar, vanilla & salt until almost doubled in mass & lightened to a yellowish-white in color, for 8 to 10 minutes, on low to middle speed.

Scrape the mixture from the sides of yours bowl using a rubber spatula. Sift the flour x 3 times & gently fold in until well incorporated.

Transfer the mixture into a sheet of plastic wrap, roll into log & cut a hole on it; placing it into the piping bag attached with a nozzle flower tips 4.6cm/1.81" x 1.18".

Pipe each cookie into 5cm wide swirls on a parchment paper lined baking tray.

Cover & place them in a freezer until firm up, for 30 minutes.

Preheat your oven to 300 F in advance. Once done; bake until the edges start to turn golden, for 20 minutes.

Let completely cool on the cooling rack before serving.

Store them in an airtight container.

Nutrition: Calories: 455, Fat: 67 g, Carbs: 12.8 g, Protein: 66.3 g, Sodium: 552 mg

Campfire S'mores

Preparation Time: 15 minutes

Cooking Time: 40 minutes

Servings: 9

Ingredients:

Graham Cracker Crust

2 cups graham cracker crumbs

¼ cup sugar

½ cup butter

½ teaspoon cinnamon

1 small package brownie mix (enough for an 8×8-inch pan), or use the brownie ingredients listed below.

Brownie Mix

½ cup flour

⅓ cup cocoa

¼ teaspoon baking powder

¼ teaspoon salt

½ cup butter

1 cup sugar

1 teaspoon vanilla

2 large eggs

S'mores Topping

9 large marshmallows

5 Hershey candy bars

4½ cups vanilla ice cream

½ cup chocolate sauce

Directions:

Preheat the oven to 350°F.

Mix together the graham cracker crumbs, sugar, cinnamon and melted butter in a medium bowl. Stir until the crumbs and sugar have combined with the butter.

Line an 8×8-inch baking dish with parchment paper. Make sure to use enough so that you'll be able to lift the baked brownies out of the dish easily. Press the graham cracker mixture into the bottom of the lined pan.

Place pan in the oven to prebake the crust a bit while you are making the brownie mixture.

Melt the butter over medium heat in a large saucepan, then stir in the sugar and vanilla. Whisk in the eggs one at a time. Then whisk in the dry ingredients, followed by the nuts. Mix until smooth. Take the crust out of the oven, pour the mixture into it, and bake for 23-25 minutes. When brownies are done, remove from oven and let cool in the pan.

After the brownies have cooled completely, lift them out of the pan using the edges of the parchment paper. Be careful not to crack or break the brownies. Cut into individual slices.

When you are ready to serve, place a marshmallow on top of each brownie and broil in the oven until the marshmallow starts to brown. You can also microwave for a couple of seconds, but you won't get the browning that you would in the broiler.

Remove from the oven and top each brownie with half of a Hershey bar. Serve with ice cream and a drizzle of chocolate sauce.

Nutrition: Calories: 187, Fat: 18.9 g, Carbs: 56.6 g, Protein: 65. 2, Sodium: 552 mg

Banana Pudding

Preparation Time: 15 minutes

Cooking Time: 1 hour and 30 minutes

Servings: 8 to 10

Ingredients:

6 cups milk

5 eggs, beaten

¼ teaspoon vanilla extract

1⅛ cups flour

1½ cups sugar

¾ pound vanilla wafers

3 bananas, peeled

8 ounces Cool Whip or 2 cups of whipped cream

Directions:

In a large saucepan, heat the milk to about 170°F.

Mix the eggs, vanilla, flour, and sugar together in a large bowl.

Very slowly add the egg mixture to the warned milk and cook until the mixture thickens to a custard consistency.

Layer the vanilla wafers to cover the bottom of a baking pan or glass baking dish. You can also use individual portion dessert dish or glasses.

Layer banana slices over the top of the vanilla wafers. Be as liberal with the bananas as you want.

Layer the custard mixture on top of the wafers and bananas. Move the pan to the refrigerator and cool for 1½ hours. When ready to serve, spread Cool Whip (or real whipped cream, if you prefer) over the top. Garnish with banana slices and wafers if desired.

Nutrition: Calories: 166, Fat: 56 g, Carbs: 78.9 g, Protein: 47.8 g, Sodium: 578 mg

Molten Chocolate Cake

Preparation Time: 1 hour 30 minutes

Cooking Time: 30 minutes

Servings: 8 to 10

Ingredients:

1 Duncan Hines fudge cake mix

3 large eggs

1 cup milk

½ cup oil

½ cup sour cream

Vanilla ice cream

Chocolate shell ice cream topping

Caramel sauce

For Magic Shell

¼ cup coconut oil

2 cups chocolate chips, semi-sweet

For Hot Fudge

1 bag semi-sweet chocolate chips (12-ounces)

4 tablespoons unsalted butter

1 can sweetened condensed milk (14-ounces)

A pinch of salt

1 teaspoon pure vanilla extract

Directions:

Stir the dry cake mix together with sour cream, eggs, milk & oil in a large bowl.

Lightly coat a large-sized cupcake pan with the nonstick spray & distribute the batter evenly approximately ¾ full. Bake as per the directions mentioned on the package.

Turn the cakes out onto their tops creating a "volcano" & let cool.

Gently cut a hole out of the middle without going clear to the bottom using a pairing or serrated knife.

Fill with cool hot fudge & then slice off the bottom circle of the piece of cake you removed and place it on the hot fudge hole like a lid.

Using a plastic wrap; cover & let chill in a fridge for 30 minutes.

Remove the cakes from freezer & reheat in the microwave for half a minute, until warm.

Top with caramel, ice cream & magic shell.

For Magic Shell

Place the chocolate along with the coconut oil in a microwave safe bowl and slowly heat for 30 second intervals until melted, stirring often.

Serve over cold ice cream & it would harden.

For Hot Fudge

Melt the entire ingredients together over medium heat in a medium saucepan.

Bring the mixture to a boil, stirring every now and then.

Continue to boil & stir for a minute or two more.

Remove the pan from heat & continue to stir for a minute.

Let the fudge sauce to cool.

Nutrition: Calories: 146, Fat: 64.5 g, Carbs: 77. 6 g, Protein: 63.8 g, Sodium: 766 mg

Paradise Pie

Preparation Time: 10 minutes

Cooking Time: 1 hour and 5 minutes

Servings: 6

Ingredients:

For Crust:

3 tablespoon granulated sugar

⅓ cup graham cracker crumbs

3 tablespoon butter

⅓ cup chocolate chips

For Filling:

½ cup flour

¼ cup coconut, shredded

¾ teaspoon baking powder

⅓ cup milk

¼ cup walnuts, crushed

1 teaspoon vanilla extract

¼ cup granulated sugar

⅓ cup semisweet chocolate chips

1 tablespoon canola oil

For Topping:

Vanilla ice cream

2 tablespoon butter

Hot fudge

¼ cup walnuts, chopped or crushed

Caramel topping

Directions:

For Crust:

Preheat oven to 350 F.

Now, in a medium-sized microwave-safe bowl; heat the butter until completely melted. When done, add in the graham cracker crumbs & sugar; mix well.

Transfer to a 1-quart casserole dish. Firmly pressing into the bottom of your dish. Evenly top with the chocolate chips.

Bake in the preheated oven until the chocolate is completely melted, for 5 minutes. Spread the melted chocolate out smoothly using a rubber spatula.

For Filling:

Combine the entire dry ingredients in a large-sized mixing bowl. Add oil, milk & vanilla; mix on low speed until completely smooth.

With mixer still on low, add in the coconut, chocolate chips & walnuts.

When mixed thoroughly, pour the filling on top of the crust.

Bake at 350 F until a wooden pick comes out clean, for 35 to 40 minutes, uncovered.

To Serve:

Spoon approximately 2 tablespoons of the butter on ovenproof plate & place in oven until the butter is completely melted.

Remove the plate from oven & place a large piece of warm pie right over the melted butter.

Top the pie with a scoop of vanilla ice cream then, top with the hot fudge & caramel toppings. Sprinkle with chopped or crushed walnuts; serve immediately & enjoy.

Nutrition: Calories: 178, Fat: 76 g, Carbs: 67.8 g, Protein: 76.9 g, Sodium:929 mg

Skillet Chocolate Chip Cookie

Preparation Time: 30 minutes

Cooking Time: 20 minutes

Servings: 8 to 10

Ingredients:

1 pouch chocolate chip cookie mix (17.5-ounce)

Hot fudge, for drizzling (store-bought or homemade)

⅓ cup chocolate chips, semi-sweet, for sprinkling

1 stick (½ cup) softened butter, unsalted

Ice cream for serving

1 large egg

Directions:

Lightly coat a 10" ovenproof skillet with the cooking spray; set aside and then Preheat oven to 350 F.

Add the cookie mix together with butter & egg to a medium-sized bowl; give the ingredients a good stir until a soft dough form.

Evenly spread the dough in skillet, smoothing with a rubber spatula.

Evenly sprinkle with the chocolate chips, pressing them down lightly using your fingertips.

Bake until the edges turn light golden brown, for 20 to 23 minutes. Ensure that you don't over bake

Place the skillet over a cooling rack & let cool for 5 minutes then drizzle with the hot fudge; serve with the ice cream.

Nutrition: Calories: 233 Fat: 87.8 g Carbs: 57.6 Protein: 65. 7 Sodium: 867 mg

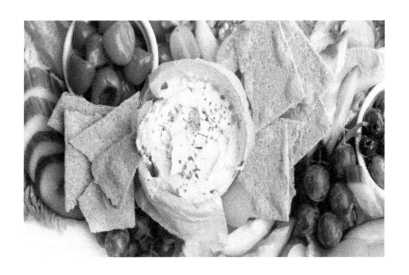

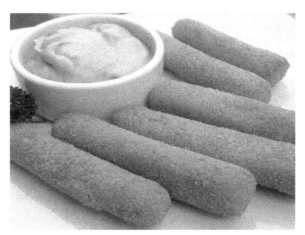

Timeless Restaurant Favorites

Starbucks® Mocha Frappuccino

Preparation Time: 10 minutes

Cooking Time: 10 minutes

Servings: 8

Ingredients

¾ cup chocolate syrup

4 cups milk

¾ cup sugar

3 cups espresso coffee

For Topping:

Chocolate syrup

Whipped cream

Directions

Prepare the coffee as per the directions provided by the manufacturer.

Mix hot coffee & sugar in a mixer until the sugar is completely dissolved, for a minute or two, on high settings.

Add chocolate syrup & milk; continue to mix for a minute more.

For easy storage, pour the mixture into a sealable container. Store in a refrigerator until ready to use.

Now, combine mix & ice (in equal proportion) in a blender & blend until smooth, on high settings & prepare the drink.

Pour the drink into separate glasses & top each glass first with the whipped cream & then drizzle chocolate syrup on the top.

Serve & enjoy!

Nutrition: Calories: 197 kcal, Protein: 4.54 g, Fat: 4.47 g, Carbohydrates: 35 g

Reese's Peanut Butter Cups

Preparation time: 15 minutes

Cooking time: 2 minutes

Chill time: 6 hours

Servings: 10

Ingredients

Salt, pinch

1½ cups peanut butter

1 cup confectioners' sugar

20 ounces milk chocolate chips

Directions

Take a medium bowl and mix the salt, peanut butter, and sugar until firm.

Place the chocolate chips in a microwave-safe bowl and microwave for 2 minutes to melt.

Grease the muffin tin with oil spray and spoon some of the melted chocolate into each muffin cup.

Take a spoon and draw the chocolate up to the edges of the muffin cups until all sides are coated.

Cool in the refrigerator for few hours.

Once chocolate is solid, spread about 1 teaspoon of peanut butter onto each cup.

Leave space to fill the edges of the cups.

Create the final layer by pouring melted chocolate on top of each muffin cup.

Let sit at room temperature until cool.

Refrigerate for a few hours until firm.

Remove the cups from the muffin tray and serve.

Nutrition: Calories 455, Total Fat 21.7 g, Carbs 59 g, Protein 9.7 g, Sodium 384 mg

Cadbury Cream Egg

Preparation time: 15 minutes

Cooking time: 2 minutes + Chill time: 3 hours 30 minutes

Servings: 6

Ingredients

⅓ cup light corn syrup

⅓ cup butter

2 teaspoons vanilla

⅓ teaspoon salt

3½ cups white sugar, ground and sifted

3 drops yellow food coloring

2 drops red food coloring

16 ounces chocolate chips, milk

3 teaspoons vegetable shortening

Directions

Take a bowl and combine corn syrup, butter, vanilla, salt and powdered sugar.

Mix all the ingredients well with a beater.

Reserve ⅓ of the mixture in a separate bowl, then add food coloring.

Chill both portions in the refrigerator for 2 hours.

Form rolls from the orange filling, about ¾-inch in diameter.

Wrap the orange rolls with white filling.

Repeat until all of the mixture is consumed.

Form in the shape of eggs.

Let sit in the refrigerator for 1 hour.

Melt the chocolate chips in the microwave.

Dip each egg roll in the melted chocolate.

Cool in the refrigerator for 30 minutes.

Once solid, serve and enjoy.

Nutrition: Calories 1004, Total Fat 34.8 g, Carbs 174 g, Protein 5.9 g, Sodium 261 mg

Loaded Potato Skins from TGI Friday's

Preparation Time: 30 minutes

Cooking Time: 7 minutes

Servings: 6

Ingredients

1 teaspoon oil

6 medium-sized potatoes

1 cup vegetable oil

8 ounces Cheddar cheese, grated

3 strips thick cut cooked bacon, diced

16 ounces sour cream

1 ripe tomato, diced

Fresh chives for serving, chopped finely

Directions:

Preheat oven to 375°F. Line a large baking sheet with parchment paper.

Using a fork, prick potatoes in a few places. Microwave for at least 10 minutes or until soft.

Halve the potatoes vertically and remove the insides of the potato until there is only ¼ inch of the potato shell left.

In a deep saucepan, heat oil to 365 °F. Deep-fry potato shells for 5 minutes, then transfer onto plate lined with paper towels.

Add cheese and diced bacon into potato shells. Place on the baking sheet prepared earlier and bake for at least 7 minutes or until cheese is fully melted.

Serve immediately with spoonful of sour cream on top or on the side. Sprinkle with diced tomatoes and chives.

Nutrition: Calories 519, Total Fat 33 g, Carbs 41 g, Protein 17 g, Sodium 361 mg

Avocado Eggrolls from The Cheesecake Factory

Preparation Time: 15 minutes

Cooking Time: 5 minutes

Servings: 8

Ingredients

Cilantro dipping sauce:

¾ cup fresh cilantro leaves, chopped

⅓ cup sour cream

2 tablespoons mayonnaise

1 garlic clove

2 tablespoons lime juice

Salt and pepper, to taste

Egg roll:

1 cup vegetable oil

3 avocados, peeled and seeded

1 Roma tomato, minced

¼ cup red onion, minced

2 tablespoons fresh cilantro leaves, diced

2 tablespoons lime juice

Salt and pepper, to taste

8 egg roll wrappers

Directions:

Mix together the ingredients for the cilantro dipping sauce in a bowl. Set aside.

Preheat a large pot with oil over medium-high heat. Oil temperature should reach 350°F and there should be enough oil to cover the rolls, about 3 to 4 inches deep

Mash avocados in a bowl. Mix in tomato, red onion, cilantro, and lime juice. Add salt and pepper, to taste.

Position avocado mixture onto the middle of an egg roll wrapper. Fold wrapper on top of mixture and roll until the mixture is fully wrapped. Secure edges of the wrapper by pressing with water using your finger. Repeat for the remaining mixture and wrappers.

Deep-fry rolls in the pot of hot oil for at least 2 minutes or until all sides are golden brown.

Remove from pot with tongs and place onto a plate lined with paper towels.

Serve with the cilantro dipping sauce on the side.

Nutrition: Calories 288, Total Fat 18 g, Carbs 28 g, Protein 6 g, Sodium 219 mg

Copycat Bloomin' Onion and Chili Sauce from Outback

Preparation Time: 20 minutes

Cooking Time: 4 minutes

Servings: 8

Ingredients

2 large sweet onions such as a Vidalia

Oil for frying

Seasoned flour:

1 cup flour

2 teaspoons paprika

1 teaspoons garlic powder

1/4 teaspoon pepper

1/8 teaspoon cayenne

Chili sauce (yields 2 1/4 cups):

1 cup mayonnaise

1 cup sour cream

1/4 cup tomato chili sauce

1/4 teaspoon cayenne

Dipping Sauce:

1/2 cup mayonnaise

2 teaspoons ketchup

2 teaspoons horseradish cream

1/4 teaspoon paprika

1/4 teaspoon salt

1/8 teaspoon dried oregano

1 dash black pepper

1 dash cayenne

Batter:

1/3 cup cornstarch

1 1/2 cups flour

2 teaspoons garlic, minced

2 teaspoons paprika

1 teaspoon salt

1 teaspoon pepper

24 ounces beer

Directions:

Preheat a large pot with oil over medium-high heat until 375 °F, not exceeding 400 °F.

In a large bowl, mix together the ingredients for the seasoned flour.

In a separate bowl, mix together the ingredients for the chili sauce.

For the dipping sauce, mix the ingredients together in a bowl and keep refrigerated.

To make the batter, combine cornstarch, flour, garlic, paprika, salt, and pepper in a bowl. Mix well.

Pour in beer to the bowl of dry ingredients. Blend well until smooth.

Chop off ¾ inches of the onion on the top. Peel, then slice until just above the bottom root end to make about 14 vertical wedges. Take out about 1 inch of petals from the inside.

Coat petals in flour, then shake off any excess. Dip in batter. Make sure the onion is well-coated.

Deep-fry for about 1 to 3 minutes, or until golden brown.

Transfer onto plate lined with paper towels to drain.

Serve with chili sauce and dipping sauce on the side.

Nutrition: Calories 404, Total Fat 12 g, Carbs 59 g, Protein 8 g, Sodium 436 mg

Deep Fried Pickles from Texas Roadhouse

Preparation Time: 10 minutes

Cooking Time: 10 minutes

Servings: 4

Ingredients

Vegetable oil, for deep frying

¼ cup flour

1¼ teaspoons Cajun seasoning, divided

¼ teaspoon oregano

¼ teaspoon basil

⅛ teaspoon cayenne pepper

Kosher salt

2 cups dill pickles, drained and sliced

¼ cup mayonnaise

1 tablespoon horseradish

1 tablespoon ketchup

Directions:

Preheat about 1½ inches oil to 375°F in a large pot.

In a separate bowl, make the coating by combining flour, 1 teaspoon Cajun seasoning, oregano, basil, cayenne pepper, and Kosher salt.

Dredge pickle slices in flour mixture. Lightly shake to remove any excess, then carefully lower into hot oil. Work in batches so as to not overcrowd the pot. Deep fry for about 2 minutes or until lightly brown.

Using a slotted spoon, transfer pickles to a plate lined with paper towels to drain.

While pickles drain and cool, add mayonnaise, horseradish, ketchup, and remaining Cajun seasoning in a bowl. Mix well.

Serve immediately with dip on the side.

Nutrition: Calories 296, Total Fat 28 g, Saturated Fat 14 g, Carbs 12 g, Sugar 4 g, Fibers 0 g, Protein 1 g, Sodium 1201 mg

The Famous Breadsticks from Olive Garden

Preparation Time: 15 minutes

Cooking Time: 15 minutes

Servings: 16

Ingredients

1½ cups plus 2 tablespoons warm water

1 package active dry yeast

4¼ cups all-purpose flour, plus more for dusting

2 tablespoons unsalted butter, softened

2 tablespoons sugar

1 tablespoon fine salt

3 tablespoons unsalted butter, melted

½ teaspoon kosher salt

¼ teaspoon garlic powder

Pinch dried oregano

Directions:

Preheat oven to 400°F. Prepare a baking tray and line it with parchment paper.

To prepare the dough, pour ¼ cup warm water in a mixing bowl. Add yeast and wait 5 minutes or until bubbles form. Combine with flour, 2 tablespoons butter, sugar, salt, and 1¼ cups and 2 tablespoons warm water. Mix for about 5 minutes or until mixture turns into dough that is a bit sticky.

Remove from bowl and transfer onto a flat surface sprinkled with flour. Knead for about 3 minutes until dough is soft and smooth. Form dough into a log that is about 2 feet long. Then, cut dough equally in 1½-inch long pieces, making 16 small pieces in total. For each piece, knead slightly and form into a breadstick that is about 7 inches long. Position breadsticks on prepared baking tray with 2-inch spaces in between each. Cover, then set aside for 45 minutes or until dough size has doubled.

Using a brush, coat breadsticks with 1½ tablespoons melted butter. Season with ¼ teaspoon salt.

Place in oven and bake for 15 minutes or until slightly golden.

As the breadsticks bake, mix remaining salt, garlic powder, and oregano in a bowl.

Remove breadsticks from oven and immediately coat with the rest of the melted butter. Season with herb mixture.

Serve warm.

Nutrition: Calories 146, Total Fat 4 g, Saturated Fat 2 g, Carbs 25 g, Sugar 2 g, Fibers 1 g, Protein 4 g, Sodium 456 mg

Hot n' Spicy Buffalo Wings from Hooters

Preparation Time: 15 minutes

Cooking Time: 12 minutes

Servings: 2

Ingredients

½ cup flour

¼ teaspoon paprika

¼ teaspoon cayenne pepper

¼ teaspoon salt

10 chicken wings

Vegetable oil, for deep frying

¼ cup butter

¼ cup Louisiana hot sauce

1 dash ground black pepper

1 dash garlic powder

Blue cheese salad dressing

Celery cut into sticks

Directions:

In a bowl, add flour, paprika, cayenne pepper, and salt. Mix well.

In a separate bowl, add chicken wings. Lightly coat with flour mixture. Make sure the coating for each wing is even. Refrigerate for at least 1 hour to keep the coating attached while frying.

To prepare, preheat about 1½-inch deep oil in deep fryer to 375°F.

In a separate small pot, heat butter, hot sauce, pepper, and garlic powder. Stir until butter is dissolved and ingredients are well mixed.

Carefully lower coated chicken wings into the hot oil. Deep fry for about 10 to 15 minutes or until wings turn partly dark brown then transfer onto a plate lined with paper towels to drain.

While the wings are still hot, transfer to a bowl and pour hot sauce mixture on top. Toss to coat all wings evenly.

Serve hot with blue cheese dressing and celery sticks.

Nutrition: Calories 867, Total Fat 63 g, Saturated Fat 26 g, Carbs 25 g, Sugar 1 g, Fibers 1 g, Protein 49 g, Sodium 1419 mg

Southwestern Eggrolls from Chili's

Preparation Time: 10 minutes

Cooking Time: 20 minutes

Servings: 4

Ingredients

1 chicken breast, boneless and skinless

8 cups plus 2 tablespoons vegetable oil, divided

2 tablespoons red bell pepper, finely chopped

2 tablespoons scallion, finely chopped

⅓ cup frozen corn

¼ cup canned black beans, rinsed and drained

2 tablespoons frozen spinach, thawed and drained

2 tablespoons pickled jalapeno peppers, chopped

½ tablespoon fresh parsley, finely chopped

½ teaspoon ground cumin

½ teaspoon chili powder

¼ plus ⅛ teaspoon salt, and more to taste

Pinch cayenne pepper

¾ cup jack cheese, grated

5 6-inch flour tortillas

1 egg, beaten

¼ cup avocado, mashed

¼ cup mayonnaise

¼ cup sour cream

1 tablespoon buttermilk

1½ teaspoons white vinegar

⅛ teaspoon dried parsley

⅛ teaspoon onion powder

Pinch dried dill weed

Pinch garlic powder

Pinch pepper, plus more to taste

2 tablespoons tomato, diced

1 tablespoon onion, diced

Directions:

Preheat grill to high heat.

Coat chicken breast with 1 tablespoon vegetable oil and season with salt and pepper. Grill for about 4 to 5 minutes on each side or until cooked through. Set aside and wait until cool. Then, chop into small cubes. Set aside.

Heat 1 tablespoon vegetable oil in a pan over medium-high heat. Stir fry red pepper and scallions for a few minutes, just enough for the vegetables to become soft. Add cooked chicken, corn, black beans, spinach, jalapeño peppers, parsley, cumin, chili powder, salt, and cayenne pepper. Cook for an additional 4 minutes. Stir until all the ingredients are mixed well.

Remove from heat and stir in cheese until melted.

Microwave tortillas wrapped in a damp cheese cloth for about 10-20 seconds on high.

For each of the five rolls, add about ⅕ chicken and vegetable mixture onto the middle part of a tortilla. Fold the edges inwards and roll tightly over the mixture. Before closing the wrap, brush egg onto the inner edge to help seal the tortilla...

Position rolls on a plate with the sealed edges facing down. Wrap everything in plastic wrap and place in the freezer. Freeze for at least 4 hours or overnight.

To prepare, preheat 8 cups oil in deep fryer to 350°F.

Prepare dipping sauce by mixing avocado, mayonnaise, sour cream, buttermilk, white vinegar, remaining salt, dried parsley, onion powder, dill weed, garlic powder, and pepper in a bowl. Set aside.

Carefully lower egg rolls in deep fryer. Cook for about 8 to 10 minutes then transfer to a plate lined with paper towels. Allow to cool for 2 minutes or until cool enough to handle.

Slice each roll diagonally lengthwise. Serve with dipping sauce garnished with tomato and onion.

Nutrition: Calories 655, Total Fat 45 g, Saturated Fat 22 g, Carbs 40 g, Sugar 2 g, Fibers 6 g, Protein 26 g, Sodium 655 mg

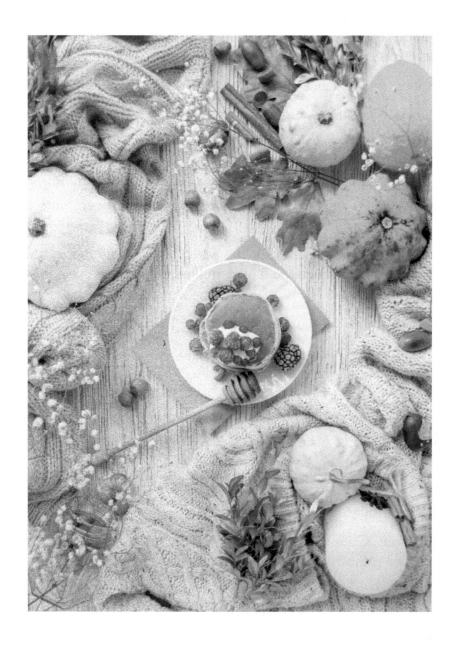

Conclusion

For meals that are scheduled to be eaten at least three days after cooking, freezing is a great option. Freezing food is safe and convenient, but it doesn't work for every type of meal. You can also freeze the ingredients for a slow cooker meal and then dump out the container into the slow cooker and leave it there. This saves a lot of time and means you can pre-prep meals up to 1-2 months in advance.

The last food safety consideration you need to make with regards to meal prepping is how you reheat food. Most people opt to microwave their meals for warming, but you can use any other conventional heating source in your kitchen as well. The reason people love the microwave for heating their meal prep meals is that it's quick and convenient.

However, you have to be careful with microwaving because over-cooking can cause food to taste bad. To combat this, cook your food in one-minute intervals and check on it between each minute. You can also help your food cook more evenly and quickly but keeping your meat cut into small pieces when you cook it. You should never put food directly from the freezer into the microwave. Let your frozen food thaw first when it's possible.

Food reheating and prep safety will become second nature over time. Meal prep can be overwhelming and require a lot of thought and patience, but it becomes a lot easier once you get used to it. Many of the mistakes are easy to avoid.

However, mistakes do happen, and as such, it's best to cook for short periods rather than longer ones, so you have less of a risk of making a mistake and needing to scrap everything you have prepared for that substantial amount of time. While it is a lot and seems complicated, meal prepping is the best way to set yourself up for success using your delicious copycat recipes. Make the meals using double the products and adjust the times; that is all it is to it!

Don't store hot food in the fridge. Keep your refrigerator at the proper temperature (should be below 40° Fahrenheit). If your refrigerator is warmer than this, it promotes the growth of bacteria. Any drastic temperature changes will cause condensation to form on the food items. You need to let your prepared food cool down in the open air - before putting it in a container and closing the lid. The increased moisture levels can open the door to bacteria growth.

Label the Containers: There are some other things you have to consider when freezing your meals. You should always label your container with the date that you put it in the freezer. You also need to double-check that your bottles, jars, or bags are each sealed tightly. If your containers aren't air-tight, your food will become freezer burnt and need to be trashed.

These recipes are the perfect additions to your daily meals. If you want affordable restaurant-style food, then here is the answer. We've got recipes from all your favorite restaurants. If you ever host a party, there are dishes in here that will make your guests ask, "Hey, what's the recipe for that chicken your served?" If you regularly cook for yourself or your family, then these simple recipes will help you elevate your meals. And if you just love having restaurant food at home, then try making some yourself—you never know, you might even be a better cook!

By cooking at home, you get to save money and time, you get to control portions, and you get to customize each meal. Remember, the recipes found here are more of a guide ultimately, you get to choose how your next meal will taste and how best to prepare it.

If you're looking for healthier substitutions for some ingredients, here is a conversion chart that you can refer to:

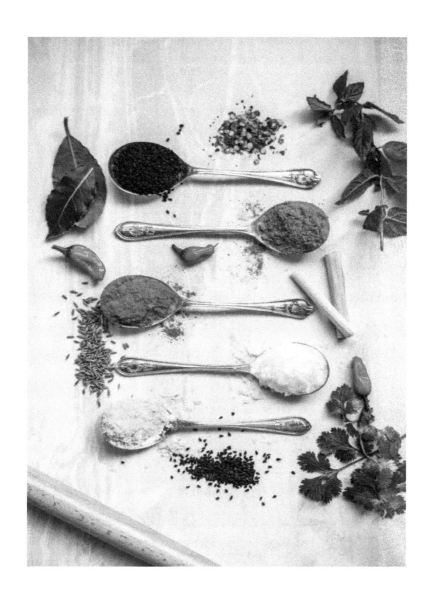

Healthier Substitutions and Conversions

White bread	Whole-wheat bread
Butter, margarine, shortening or oil to prevent sticking	Cooking spray or nonstick pans
Cream cheese	Fat-free or low-fat cream cheese, fat-free ricotta cheese
Cheese	Low-fat or fat-free cheese
Eggs	Two egg whites or $\frac{1}{4}$ cup egg substitute for each whole egg
White flour	Whole-wheat flour for half of the called-for all-purpose flour
Ground beef	Extra-lean or lean ground beef, chicken or turkey breast
Whole milk	Evaporated skim milk, reduced-fat or fat-free milk
Pasta	Whole-wheat pasta
White rice	Brown rice, wild rice, bulgur, or pearl barley
Salad dressing	Fat-free or reduced-calorie dressing or flavored vinegars
Salt	Herbs, spices, fruit juices or salt-free seasoning mixes or herb blends
Syrup	Pureed fruit, such as applesauce, or low-calorie, sugar-free syrup

Standard U.S./Metric Measurement Conversions

VOLUME CONVERSIONS	
U.S. Volume Measure	Metric Equivalent
1/8 teaspoon	0.5 milliliters
1/4 teaspoon	1 milliliters
1/2 teaspoon	2 milliliters
1 teaspoon	5 milliliters
1/2 tablespoon	7 milliliters
1 tablespoon (3 teaspoons)	15 milliliters
2 tablespoons (1 fluid ounce)	30 milliliters
1/4 cup (4 tablespoons)	60 milliliters
1/3 cup	90 milliliters
1/2 cup (4 fluid ounces)	125 milliliters
2/3 cup	160 milliliters
3/4 cup (6 fluid ounces)	180 milliliters
1 cup (16 tablespoons)	250 milliliters
1 pint (2 cups)	500 milliliters
1 quart (4 cups)	1 liter (about)

WEIGHT CONVERSIONS	
U.S. Weight Measure	Metric Equivalent
½ ounce	15 grams
1 ounce	30 grams
2 ounces	60 grams
3 ounces	85 grams
¼ pound (4 ounces)	115 grams
½ pound (8 ounces)	225 grams
¾ pound (12 ounces)	340 grams
1 pound (16 ounces)	454 grams

OVEN TEMPERATURE CONVERSIONS	
Degrees Fahrenheit	Degrees Celsius
200 degrees F	100 degrees C
250 degrees F	120 degrees C
275 degrees F	140 degrees C
300 degrees F	150 degrees C
325 degrees F	160 degrees C
350 degrees F	180 degrees C
375 degrees F	190 degrees C
400 degrees F	200 degrees C
425 degrees F	220 degrees C
450 degrees F	230 degrees C

Hopefully, these recipes have given you a few tips and tricks on how to recreate your favorite restaurant dishes at home. The book is meant to give you some motivation and inspiration to cook these meals in the comforts of your own home.

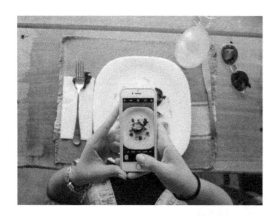

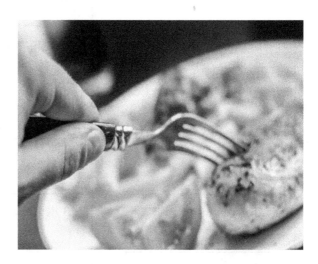

MELISSA POT

COPYCAT
RESTAURANT FAVORITES

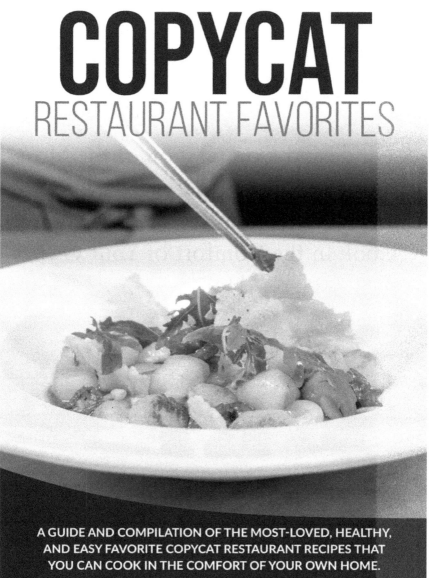

A GUIDE AND COMPILATION OF THE MOST-LOVED, HEALTHY, AND EASY FAVORITE COPYCAT RESTAURANT RECIPES THAT YOU CAN COOK IN THE COMFORT OF YOUR OWN HOME.

COPYCAT RESTAURANT FAVORITES

A Guide and Compilation of the Most-Loved, Healthy, and Easy Favorite Copycat Restaurant Recipes that you can Cook in the Comfort of Your Own Home

Melissa Pot

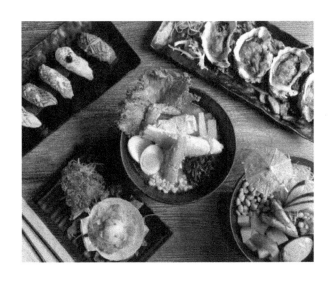

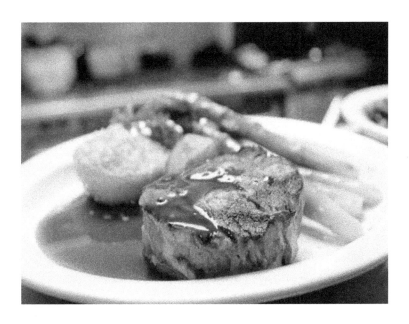

Introduction

With a recession scare creeping across the economy and your budget likely getting a very tight squeeze, you're probably looking for some way to stretch it out and make it last. Do you believe that Copycat Recipes will help you recover any, perhaps a whole bunch of dollars in your budget?

It will certainly do that, and once you look at it, it's simple math. In making copycat recipes you'll not only save a lot on the expense of' eating out' but also on gas, and that's a huge bonus. Just to offer a quick example, and these are very conservative figures, if you eat out just twice a week and spend around $45 in the sum of each dinner out, that is $360 a month. Note, this doesn't even include the cost of driving to your favorite locations. Many people probably spend a lot more than eating out each month, depending on where you are going and how many people you are shopping for. Do you see how much money you can save by making these homemade meals?

The question you might ask is, how can you cook a dish or meal from scratch, with your own ingredients that will taste as good as what you can find at your favorite restaurant or eating establishment? It is easy when you can get your hands on a strong Copycat Recipes set or source.

These are reverse engineered recipes that were passed down from some of the original chefs who created the popular meals in the restaurants. It helps you to design and recreate recipes of previously hidden dishes for use and enjoyment in your home. So close, as a matter of fact, that you wouldn't be able to tell the difference between the one you cooked and the one from the restaurant!

So, by accessing Copycat Recipes, you can basically make your family super happy by serving their favorite meals whenever they want, and put a bunch of money back into your pocket every month by wiping out your monthly "eating out" budget!

If you are having a party, you can make a copycat restaurant recipe that will have your guests swearing you purchased it from the restaurant that made the dish famous. You can enjoy the attention your cooking will bring when you decide to make a copycat restaurant recipe for your next party or potluck dinner.

Just because you cook your own food doesn't mean it can't be as delicious as a five-star restaurant; all you need are a few simple tools. You don't have to be a master chef to cook like one, either. The equipment needed to prepare the recipes in this book are broken into appliances, cooking gadgets, cookware, and bakeware. You will also learn the terms and techniques needed to make a wonderful restaurant-quality meal.

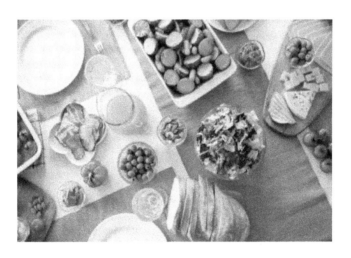

The Essential Kitchen Gear

Appliances

These appliances will provide the greatest convenience and versatility in your kitchen:

- Electric mixer — A portable handheld mixer will do well for all of the recipes in this book.

- Blender — This kitchen helper cuts time instantly by blending, chopping, and puréeing foods.

- Deep fryer — A small Fry Daddy is the best at regulating the temperature of the cooking oil when deep frying meats or vegetables.

- George Foreman Indoor Grill — This is a great time saver in the kitchen when grilling any kind of meat, since both sides cook at once.

- Microwave oven — As ubiquitous as they are, you can rely on them for quick thawing and heating jobs in the kitchen.

Cooking Gadgets

A good cook knows that a good-quality set of knives can accomplish more in the kitchen than any electronic device. These are the knives that you will need:

- A chef's knife that has a broad, tapered shape, which can easily be rocked over ingredients.

- A bread knife, which has a serrated edge that makes it perfect for cutting through crusts.

- A paring knife has a short blade that is used for peeling, trimming, coring, and seeding vegetables.

Cooking in the kitchen can be fun, but it is a spot for potential accidents. There are some basic safety rules you should follow to make your cooking experience more enjoyable: The kitchen is not the place to go barefoot; it is important to understand your tools and how to handle them properly; read the instructions on how to use your appliances.

Other Tools

Other tools needed in food preparation include:

- Bottle opener

- Can opener

- Colander

- Cutting board

- Grater

- Long-handled forks, spoons, and spatulas

- Meat mallet

- Pizza cutter

- Rolling pin

- Set of measuring cups

- Set of measuring spoons

- Set of mixing bowls

Cookware

You'll also need the following pieces of cookware:

- Saucepans with lids (small, medium, and large)

- Stockpot (large enough to make soup for your family)

- Cast-iron skillet (for using in the oven)

- 12" nonstick skillet

Bakeware

Don't forget these necessary pieces of bakeware:

- Baking sheets

- Casserole dishes (small, medium, and large)

- Muffin pan

- Rectangular sheet cake pan

- Roasting pan with a rack

- Pizza pan

Stocking the Pantry

Cooking is much easier when you know what you've already got on hand and aren't running to the grocery store every time you want to fix a meal. Having a well-stocked pantry is a cook's secret weapon. Here is a list of basic ingredients that should be in your pantry. Of course, you can adjust items on the list to suit your family's likes and dislikes.

Herbs and Spices

If you've spent any time in the spice aisle at the supermarket lately, you know how expensive spices are. A little bottle will set you back a couple of bucks. Therefore, it is recommended that you buy seasoning blends. Some of the most common and widely used flavors are:

- Barbecue seasoning, which contains a variety of spices that are good sprinkled onto meat before grilling, roasting or broiling.

- Cajun seasoning is a blend of red pepper, garlic, onion, salt, and pepper used to add a hot taste to any dish.

- Italian seasoning is a favorite mix of basil and oregano useful in most pasta dishes.

- Lemon pepper seasoning adds flavor to poultry and vegetables.

- Mexican seasoning contains a mixture of peppers, garlic, salt, and cumin suitable for tacos, fajitas, and enchiladas.

A great way to stock your pantry with spices is to buy one or two new ones each time you go shopping and buy fresh herbs only when needed.

Sauces

Sauces are a great way to add flavor to your dishes. Here are some sauces you should have on hand in your kitchen:

- Barbecue sauce

- Chili sauce

- Hot pepper sauce

- Olive oil

- Packages of dried onion soup mix

- Packages of salad dressing mix

- Soy sauce

- Soups in a can (cream of mushroom, chicken, celery)

- Steak sauce

- Sweet and sour sauce

- Teriyaki sauce

- Vinegar (red, rice, and balsamic)

- Wine (red and white suitable, for drinking)

- Worcestershire sauce

Basic Grocery Items

You also need some essential grocery items, things you will find yourself using over and over in myriad recipes. These kitchen basics include:

- Beans (a variety of canned and dried)

- Bread crumbs

- Bullion cubes and powders

- Cooking oil

- Crackers (a variety)

- Croutons

- Meats (canned tuna, chicken, crab, and clams)

- Olives (black and green)

- Pastas (a mixed variety)

- Rice (white, long grain, wild, brown)

- Salsa

- Tomatoes (a variety of canned)

- Tomato paste

- Tomato sauce

Baking Items

To bake like the best restaurants, you need to keep some baking basics in your pantry, including:

- Baking mix

- Baking powder

- Baking soda

- Brown sugar

- Confectioners' sugar

- Cocoa powder

- Cornstarch

- Flavored chips (chocolate, peanut butter, caramel)

- Flour

- Honey

- Nuts (a variety)

- Pancake mix

- Sugar

- Sweetened condensed milk

- Vegetable shortening

- Yeast

For Desserts

To create many restaurant-inspired desserts, you should have the following on hand:

- Applesauce

- Canned fruits

- Cake mixes, brownies, and frostings

- Fixings for ice cream sundaes

- Puddings

In the Refrigerator

Keep these items handy in the fridge so you can whip up your favorite copycat recipes without having to run out to the store. Make sure to have:

- Butter or margarine

- Cheeses (a good variety)

- Cream

- Eggs

- Ketchup

- Milk

- Mayonnaise

- Mustard

- Salad dressings

- Salad fixings (a variety of fresh vegetables)

- Sour cream

In the Freezer

There are a few items that, while you won't use them every day, you'll still want to keep stocked in your freezer. They include:

- Baguettes

- Boneless, skinless chicken breasts

- Bread and pizza dough

- Ground beef

- Steaks

- Stew meat

- Vegetables (broccoli, spinach, sliced green peppers)

With all these things on hand, you can put together a tasty and beautifully presented restaurant copycat meal in just a few minutes. The only thing you'll have to worry about is which recipe you want to try next.

Choosing Ingredients

Cooking from scratch always tastes better. Restaurant chefs seek out the freshest ingredients they can find and so should you. Skip the prepackaged items whenever you can. Generic brands may offer a lower price, but be careful to check out the quality and flavor — you may not be satisfied with the final taste of the dish. By upgrading your choices, you can turn an ordinary meal into something special. For example, instead of using plain iceberg lettuce try romaine or a spring mix, and don't settle for boring American cheese. Experiment and try new flavors.

Meats

Red meats should have a rosy bloom and poultry should look plump and moist. Meat packages should be firmly wrapped, with no leaking or excess moisture. Check expiration dates and package labeling to make sure that the meat is fresh and has been handled properly. Refrigerate meats as soon as they are purchased. Price is not always a reflection of quality; don't assume that the most expensive meat is the best.

Chicken

You can buy a whole chicken or in any variety of precut packages. The key to cooking with chicken is to be careful to avoid cross contamination and the risk of salmonella. Wash your hands and the chicken before cooking. Keep the uncooked chicken away from everything else on the kitchen counter. Use a separate cutting board and knife just for the uncooked chicken and do not use those same utensils for anything else. Clean anything the chicken touches thoroughly. If you follow these precautions, cooking with chicken is perfectly safe.

Beef

According to the USDA, ground beef cannot contain more than 30 percent fat by weight, so all of the packages will state their fat content. Get to know your butcher, and when London Broil or other roasts go on sale, have him grind it up for you to get premium ground beef at a reduced price.

How do you tell a great steak from a regular steak? The things to look for when buying a steak are the grade and the cut. Grade refers to the age of the animal and the marbling of the meat. The USDA grades the best steaks as prime, followed by choice and select. When selecting a steak, always take a look at the marbling or streaks of fat running through the meat. You want thin streaks that produce the best flavor. Cuts of steak are taken from different sections of the animal: The rib produces rib roast, back ribs, and rib eye steaks; the short loin produces the tastiest steaks like the T-bone, Porter-house, New York Strip, and the best cut of tenderloin.

ESSENTIAL

Always thaw meat in the refrigerator for maximum safety. Also, look for the safe handling label on packages of raw meat. It will tell you how to safely store, handle, and prepare meat and poultry.

Pork

All pork found in retail stores is inspected by the USDA. When buying pork, look for cuts with a relatively small amount of fat over the outside and with meat that is firm and grayish pink in color. For the best flavor, the meat should have a small amount of marbling. There are four basic cuts into which all other cuts are separated: the leg, side, loin, and shoulder. From those cuts, you get the bacon, ground pork for sausage, ribs, roasts, chops, and ham.

Fish

Knowing how to choose fresh fish is a skill all cooks should have. A fresh fish should smell like clean water. The eyes of the fish should be bright and clear and the gills should be a rich bright red. If it smells bad or looks discolored, don't buy it.

Fruits

Look for tenderness, plumpness, and bright color when choosing your fruit. Fruits should be heavy for their size and free of bruises, cuts, mildew, mold, or any other blemishes.

- Bananas are sold in any stage of ripeness and should be stored at room temperature.

- Berries should separate easily from their stems. Keep them refrigerated.

- Melons that have a sweet aromatic scent should be chosen. A strong smell indicates that they are overripe.

- Oranges, grapefruits, and lemons are sold when they are ripe. You may store them in the refrigerator for 2–3 weeks.

Vegetables

Take the time to inspect each vegetable before you buy. Look for crisp, plump, and brightly colored vegetables. Avoid the ones that are shriveled, bruised, moldy, or blemished.

- Asparagus should have straight stalks that are compact, with closed tips.

- Beans that are brightly colored and crisp are the best to select.

- Broccoli heads that are light green and yellowing should be avoided.

- Cabbage should have bright leaves without brown spots.

- Cauliflower with withered leaves and brown spots should not be chosen.

- Celery stalks should have firm crisp ribs.

- Cucumbers should be firm and not have soft spots.

- Peas that are shriveled or have brown spots should be avoided.

- Peppers that are crisp and bright colored should be chosen.

- Spinach leaves should be crisp and free of moisture.

Food Presentation

Whenever you go to an awesome restaurant, the vibes around that place become as important as the quality of the food served in determining whether or not you have a fulfilling experience. Remember that food presentation and table setting is of utmost value when serving a restaurant copycat meal.

Garnishes

The ingredients in the dish can pull double duty as garnishes. Save some fresh chopped herbs required in the dish to add just before plating. Use diced tomatoes or green onions on top of a dish. Shredded or shaved cheeses add a nice touch to almost any dish.

Plating

There are several types of plating techniques restaurants use, including:

- Pie style is where the plate is divided with a section for the protein, starch, and vegetables.

- The half-and-half style of plating is where the main dish is on one side of the plate with the accompaniments located on the other.

- Vertical plating is where you build the plate upward, usually with the protein on the bottom and the side dishes on top.

- Family style plating is where the food is served on large platters meant to be shared.

Soup is such an inexpensive food to make at home. Why not splurge on some fancy oven-proof soup bowls to give a meal that special restaurant feeling with melted cheese on top?

Presenting Desserts

To showcase your beautifully created restaurant desserts, serve them in individual glass drinking glasses. A small wine glass layered with cake and ice cream or fruit and yogurt makes a nice presentation. Dessert shots are all the rage in the restaurants right now. Small sweet treats is a trend that's found its way onto dessert carts all over America. Little mini parfaits, sundaes, and layered cakes in shot glasses can easily be adapted for the home cook. It is time to raid your bar and fill those shot glasses with dessert. Small juice glasses also work well serving small-sized after-dinner treats.

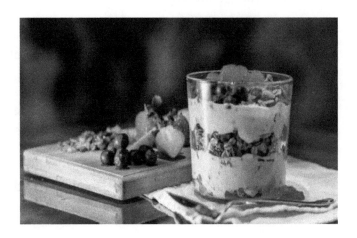

Breakfast

IHOP's Buttermilk Pancake

Preparation time: 5 minutes

Cooking time: 8 minutes

Servings: 8 to 10

Ingredients:

1¼ cups all-purpose flour

1 teaspoon baking soda

1 teaspoon baking powder

1¼ cups granulated sugar

1 pinch salt

1 egg

1¼ cups buttermilk

¼ cup cooking oil

Directions:

Preheat your pan by leaving it over medium heat while you are preparing the pancake batter.

Take all of your dry ingredients and mix them together.

Take all of your wet ingredients and mix them together.

Carefully combine the dry mixture into the wet mixture until everything is mixed together completely.

Melt some butter in your pan.

Slowly pour batter into the pan until you have a 5-inch circle.

Flip the pancake when its edges seem to have hardened.

Cook the other side of the pancake until it is golden brown.

Repeat steps six through eight until your batter is finished.

Serve with softened butter and maple syrup.

Nutrition: Calories 180.1, Total Fat 7.9 g, Carbs 23.2 g, Protein 4.1 g, Sodium 271.6 mg

McDonald's Breakfast Burrito

Preparation time: 10 minutes

Cooking time: 16 minutes

Servings: 10

Ingredients:

½ pound bulk sausage, cooked, crumbled

10 eggs, scrambled

1 medium tomato, diced

1 small onion, diced

3 tablespoons canned green chili, diced

Some salt and pepper

10 flour tortillas, warm

10 slices American cheese, halved

Some salsa

Some sour cream

Directions:

Mix the first six ingredients together in a medium-sized bowl.

Butter a non-stick pan over medium heat.

Pour the mixture into the pan and then cook until the egg is cooked the way you like.

When the mixture has reached your desired consistency, take it off the heat.

Lay out the tortillas and start assembling your burritos by placing one-tenth of the mixture in each of the tortillas.

Place the cheese on top of the egg mixture, then roll up the tortilla to make the burrito.

Garnish the roll with salsa and sour cream and serve.

Nutrition: Calories 270.1, Total Fat 14.8 g, Carbs 18.2 g, Protein 15.2 g, Sodium 525.3 mg

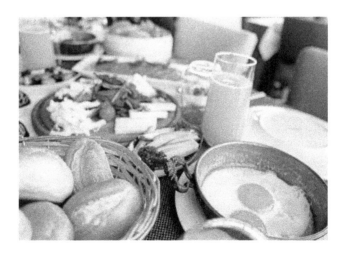

Starbucks's Marble Pound Cake

Preparation Time: 10 minutes

Cooking Time: 1 hour 30 minutes

Servings: 16

Ingredients:

4½ cups cake flour

2 teaspoons baking powder

⅛ teaspoon salt

6 ounces semisweet chocolate, finely chopped

2 cups unsalted butter, softened

3 cups granulated sugar

1 tablespoon vanilla

1 lemon, grated for zest

10 large eggs

2 tablespoons orange liquor OR milk

Directions:

Assemble your ingredients, and then:

a)   Preheat the oven to 350°F;

b)   Grease a 10×4-inch tube pan;

c)   Line the pan's bottom with greased wax paper; and

d)   Flour the entire pan.

Sift together the cake flour, baking powder, and salt in a medium-sized bowl—this is your dry mixture.

Melt the chocolate in a medium-sized bowl, then beat in the butter. When the mixture is smooth, beat in the sugar, lemon zest, and vanilla until the liquid mixture is uniform.

When the mixture is fully beaten, beat in the eggs, two at a time, until the mixture looks curdled.

Pour half of your dry mixture into your liquid mixture and mix until blended.

Add the orange liquor and the rest of the dry mixture. Continue beating the mixture.

When the mixture is blended, use a spatula to start folding it—this is your batter.

Set aside 4 cups of the batter. Whisk the melted chocolate into the remaining batter.

Now that you have a light batter and a dark batter, place the batter into the tube pan by the spoonful, alternating between the two colors.

When the pan is full, shake it slightly to level the batter. Run a knife through the batter to marble it.

Place the pan in the oven and bake for an hour and 15 minutes. To test if the cake is done, poke it with a toothpick. If there are still some moist crumbs on the toothpick when you take it out, then the cake is done.

Remove the cake from the pan and leave it to rest overnight.

Nutrition: Calories 582.1, Total Fat 32 g, Carbs 69.6 g, Protein 8.6 g, Sodium 114.8 mg

IHOP's Scrambled Egg

Preparation Time: 5 minutes

Cooking Time: 5 minutes

Servings: 4

Ingredients:

¼ cup pancake mix

1–2 tablespoons butter 6 large eggs

Salt and pepper, to taste

Directions:

Thoroughly beat the pancake mix and the eggs together until no lumps or clumps remain.

Butter a pan over medium heat.

When the pan is hot enough, pour the egg mixture in the middle of the pan.

Add the salt and pepper and let the mixture sit for about a minute.

When the egg starts cooking, start pushing the edges of the mixture toward the middle of the pan. Continue until the entire mixture is cooked.

Serve and enjoy.

Nutrition: Calories 870, Total Fat 54 g, Carbs 9 g, Protein 69 g, Sodium 34.9 mg

McDonald's' Fruit and Yogurt Parfait

Preparation Time: 5 minutes

Cooking Time: n/a

Servings: 10

Ingredients:

6 ounces vanilla yogurt, divided into 3

4-6 strawberries, sliced

¼ cup blueberries, fresh or frozen; divided into 2

¼ cup pecans, chopped; divided into 2

Directions:

Place 2 ounces of vanilla yogurt at the bottom of a cup, followed by 2-3 strawberries and ⅛ cup each of blueberries and pecans.

Place another layer of yogurt, strawberries, blueberries, and pecans on top of the first layer.

Finish off the parfait with the remaining yogurt—you can garnish it with more fruits if you like.

Nutrition: Calories 328.9, Total Fat 25.4 g, Carbs 20.7 g, Protein 9 g, Sodium 79.7 mg

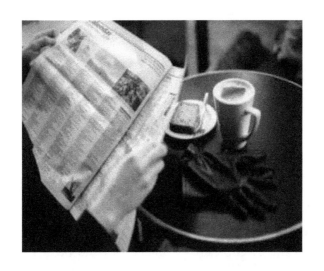

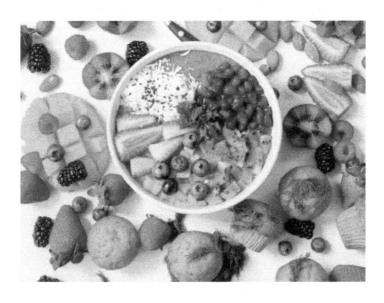

226

Panera Bread's Cinnamon Crunch Bagel

Preparation Time: 1 hour

Cooking Time: 25 minutes

Servings: 8

Ingredients:

Bread:

1¼ cups warm water, between 110 to 120°F

1 tablespoon yeast

1 tablespoon salt

4 tablespoons honey, divided

1½ cups whole wheat pastry flour

½ tablespoon cinnamon

1¾ cups bread flour

¾ cup white chocolate chips

Cornmeal, for sprinkling

4¼ quarts water

Topping:

¼ cup granulated sugar

¼ cup packed brown sugar

1 tablespoon cinnamon

⅓ cup coconut oil

Directions:

Activate the yeast by mixing it with the warm water and setting it aside for 10 minutes.

Add in 3 tablespoons of the honey, the salt, the pastry flour, and the cinnamon. Mix all the ingredients together with a dough mixer or wooden spoon. After a minute of mixing, or when the flour is fully incorporated, scrape the sides of the bowl and mix again for another few minutes.

Let the dough rest for 5 minutes—if lumps form, stir the batter to break them apart.

Add in half a cup of bread flour and start kneading. Keep adding the bread flour half a cup at a time until it is finished, while kneading the dough to distribute the flour throughout.

After about seven minutes of kneading, add in the white chocolate chips and continue kneading to completely incorporate the chips into the mixture.

Cover the bowl with a towel and leave the dough to rest for one hour.

After an hour, flour a flat surface where you can place your dough. Transfer the dough from its bowl to the floured surface and punch it down.

Cut the dough into 8 equal pieces. Roll them into ropes. Let the dough rest again, for 3 to 4 minutes.

Form a circle with each piece of dough, twisting the ends securely together. Sprinkle a baking sheet with cornmeal and place the dough circles on the sheet. Cover with a towel and let rest for 10 to 15 minutes.

While the dough is resting, prepare your materials by:

(1) Bringing the water to a boil. When the water is boiling, add the remaining 1 tablespoon of honey. Keep the water at a low boil;

(2) Preheat the oven to 450°F;

(3) Line a baking sheet with parchment or wax paper; and

(4) Mix the topping ingredients (except the oil) together.

After 15 minutes, place a few dough circles into the boiling water. Leave them to cook for 50 seconds on each side. When the bagels have boiled, transfer them to the baking sheet using a slotted spoon so as to drain off the water.

When all the bagels have boiled, brush each one with coconut oil and sprinkle with the sugar mixture.

Bake your bagels for 20 to 25 minutes, then transfer them to a wire rack to let them cool.

Nutrition: Calories 463, Total Fat 16 g, Carbs 71 g, Protein 6 g, Sodium 296 mg

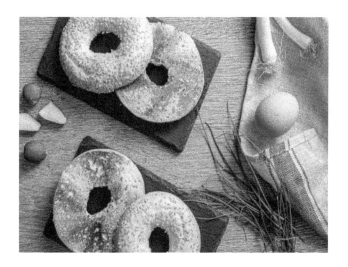

Starbucks's Chocolate Cinnamon

Bread

Preparation Time: 15 minutes

Cooking Time: 1 hour

Servings: 16

Ingredients:

Bread:

1½ cups unsalted butter

3 cups granulated sugar

5 large eggs

2 cups flour

1¼ cups processed cocoa

1 tablespoon ground cinnamon

1 teaspoon salt

½ teaspoon baking powder

½ teaspoon baking soda

¼ cup water

1 cup buttermilk

1 teaspoon vanilla extract

Topping:

¼ cup granulated sugar

½ teaspoon cinnamon

½ teaspoon processed cocoa

⅛ teaspoon ginger, ground

⅛ teaspoon cloves, ground

Directions:

Before cooking:

a)   Preheat the oven to 350°F;

b)   Grease two 9×5×3 loaf pans; and

c)   Line the bottoms of the pans with wax paper.

Cream the sugar by beating it with the butter.

Beat the eggs into the mixture one at a time.

Sift the flour, cocoa, cinnamon, salt, baking powder, and baking soda into a large bowl.

In another bowl, whisk together the water, buttermilk, and vanilla.

Make a well in the dry mixture and start pouring in the wet mixtures a little at a time, while whisking.

When the mixture starts becoming doughy, divide it in two and transfer it to the pans.

Mix together all the topping ingredients and sprinkle evenly on top of the mixture in both pans.

Bake for 50 to 60 minutes, or until the bread has set.

Nutrition: Calories 370, Total Fat 14 g, Carbs 59 g, Protein 7 g, Sodium 270 mg

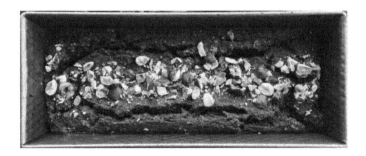

Starbucks's Lemon Loaf

Preparation Time: 15 minutes

Cooking Time: 45 minutes

Servings: 8

Ingredients:

Bread:

1½ cups flour

½ teaspoon baking soda

½ teaspoon baking powder

½ teaspoon salt

1 cup sugar

3 eggs, room temperature

2 tablespoons butter, softened

1 teaspoon vanilla extract sep

⅓ cup lemon juice

½ cup oil

Icing:

1 cup + 1 tablespoon powdered sugar

2 tablespoons milk

½ teaspoon lemon extract

Directions:

Get your baking materials ready by:

a)   Preheating your oven to 350°F;

b)   Greasing and flouring a 9×5×3 loaf pan; and

c)   Lining pan's bottom with wax paper.

Mix the first four ingredients in a large bowl—this is your dry mixture.

Beat the eggs, butter, vanilla, and lemon juice together in a medium bowl until the mixture becomes smooth. This is your wet mixture.

Make a well in the middle of the dry mixture and pour the wet mixture into the well.

Mix everything together with a whisk or your hand mixer. Add the oil. Do not stop mixing until everything is fully blended and smooth.

Pour the batter into the pan and bake it for 45 minutes—the bread is ready when you can stick a toothpick into it and it comes out clean.

While the bread is baking, make the icing by mixing the icing ingredients in a small bowl using a whisk or hand mixer until smooth.

When the bread is done baking, place it on a cooling rack and leave it for at least 20 minutes to cool.

When the bread is cool enough, pour the icing over the top. Wait for the icing to set before slicing.

Nutrition: Calories 425.2, Total Fat 18.7 g, Carbs 60 g, Protein 5 g, Sodium 310.8 mg

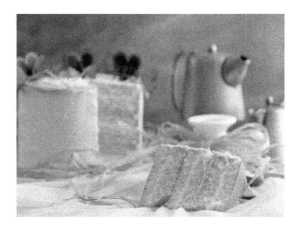

Waffle House's Waffle

Preparation Time: 5 minutes

Cooking Time: 20 minutes

Servings: 6

Ingredients:

1½ cups all-purpose flour

1 teaspoon salt

½ teaspoon baking soda

1 egg

½ cup + 1 tablespoon granulated white sugar

2 tablespoons butter, softened

2 tablespoons shortening

½ cup half-and-half

½ cup milk

¼ cup buttermilk

¼ teaspoon vanilla

Directions:

Prepare the dry mixture by sifting the flour into a bowl and mixing it with the salt and baking soda.

In a medium bowl, lightly beat an egg. When the egg has become frothy, beat in the butter, sugar, and shortening. When the mixture is thoroughly mixed, beat in the half-and-half, vanilla, milk, and buttermilk. Continue beating the mixture until it is smooth.

While beating the wet mixture, slowly pour in the dry mixture, making sure to mix thoroughly and remove all the lumps.

Chill the batter overnight (optional, but recommended; if you can't chill the mixture overnight, leave it for at least 15 to 20 minutes).

Take the batter out of the refrigerator. Preheat and grease your waffle iron.

Cook each waffle for three to four minutes. Serve with butter and syrup.

Nutrition: Calories 313.8, Total Fat 12.4 g, Carbs 45 g, Protein 5.9 g, Sodium 567.9 mg

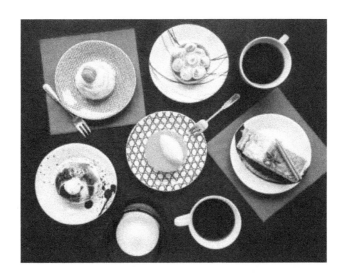

Mimi's Café Santa Fé Omelet

Preparation Time: 10 minutes

Cooking Time: 10 minutes

Servings: 1

Ingredients:

Chipotle Sauce:

1 cup marinara or tomato sauce

¾ cup water

½ cup chipotle in adobo sauce

1 teaspoon kosher salt

Omelet:

1 tablespoon onions, diced

1 tablespoon jalapeños, diced

2 tablespoons cilantro, chopped

2 tablespoons tomatoes, diced

¼ cup fried corn tortillas, cut into strips

3 eggs, beaten

2 slices cheese

1 dash of salt and pepper

Garnish:

2 ounces chipotle sauce, hot

¼ cup fried corn tortillas, cut into strips

1 tablespoon sliced green onions

1 tablespoon guacamole

Directions:

Melt some butter in a pan over medium heat, making sure to coat the entire pan.

Sauté the jalapeños, cilantro, tomatoes, onions, and tortilla strips for about a minute.

Add the eggs, seasoning them with salt and pepper and stirring occasionally.

Flip the omelet when it has set. Place the cheese on the top half.

When the cheese starts to become melty, fold the omelet in half and transfer to a plate.

Garnish the omelet with chipotle sauce, guacamole, green onions, and corn tortillas.

Nutrition: Calories 519, Total Fat 32 g, Carbs 60 g, Protein 14 g, Sodium 463 mg

Appetizers

Southwestern Egg Rolls

Preparation Time: 10 minutes

Cooking Time: 10 minutes

Servings: 6

Ingredients:

For Smoked Chicken **Ingredients:**

8 ounces chicken breast

1 teaspoon vegetable oil or olive oil

Egg Roll filling:

½ cup canned black beans, rinsed & drained

¼ cup red bell peppers, minced

2 teaspoons pickled jalapeno peppers, chopped

½ cup frozen corn

8 flour tortillas (7" each)

¼ cup spinach, frozen, thawed & drained

1 teaspoon taco seasoning

¾ cup Monterey jack cheese, shredded

1 tablespoon vegetable oil or olive oil

¼ cup green onions, minced

Avocado Ranch Ingredients

½ cup milk

1 package Ranch dressing mix

½ cup mayonnaise

¼ cup fresh avocados, smashed (approximately half of an avocado)

For Toppings:

1 tablespoon onions, chopped

2 tablespoons tomatoes, chopped

Directions:

For Chicken Breast:

Preheat grill over moderate heat. Generously season the chicken pieces with black pepper and salt. Brush the chicken breast with vegetable or olive oil. Grill over the preheated hot grill; cook for 5 to 7 minutes per side. Chop the chicken into small pieces; set aside until ready to use.

For Egg roll filling:

Sauté the red pepper for a couple of minutes, until just become tender. Add the corn, green onion, pickled jalapenos, and black beans to the mixture. Add in the taco seasoning; continue to cook until heated through.

Place equal amounts of filing, equal portions of chicken into the tortillas & top with the cheese. Fold in the ends & tightly roll them up. Secure your wrapped tortillas with toothpicks.

For Egg Rolls

Fill a large pot with vegetable oil (enough to cover the bottom by 4") and then heat it over moderate heat. Once hot; deep fry the egg rolls for 7 to 8 minutes in total, until turn golden brown. When done; immediately remove them from the hot oil & arrange them on a wire rack.

For Avocado Ranch Dressing

Prepare the Ranch dressing mix with ½ cup of buttermilk & ½ cup mayonnaise. Add approximately ¼ cup of the mashed avocado into the mixture. Add the mixture in a blender and pulse on high for a minute, until blended well.

Nutrition: Calories: 123, Fat: 23 g, Carbs: 46 g, Protein: 16 g, Sodium: 87

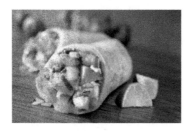

Skillet Queso

Preparation Time: 5 minutes

Cooking Time: 15 minutes

Servings: 4

Ingredients:

16 ounce box Velveeta cheese; cut into cubes

½ teaspoon ground cayenne pepper

2 teaspoons paprika

1 cups milk

15 ounce can Hormel Chili No Beans

Juice of 1 medium lime, freshly squeezed (approximately 1 tablespoon)

4 teaspoons chili powder

½ teaspoon ground cumin

Directions:

Over medium heat in a medium saucepan; combine the cheese together with the leftover ingredients. Cook for a couple of minutes, until the cheese melts completely, stirring frequently to prevent sticking.

Serve the queso with tortilla chips and enjoy.

Nutrition: Calories:533, Fat:25 g, Carbs: 47 g, Protein: 12 g, Sodium:1129 mg

White Spinach Queso

Preparation Time: 5 minutes

Cooking Time: 10 minutes

Servings: 12

Ingredients:

2 tablespoons flour

8 ounces white American cheese

2 cups baby spinach leaves, fresh

¾ cup whole milk

2 tablespoons butter

½ teaspoon garlic powder

2 cups Jack cheese

1 tablespoon canola oil

Optional **Ingredients:**

Queso fresco crumbles

Pico de Gallo salsa

Guacamole

Directions:

Set your oven to broil. Now, over medium high heat in a large, cast iron skillet; heat the canola oil until hot. Add and cook the spinach until just wilted; immediately remove from the hot pan.

Add butter to the hot pan and then add the flour, stir well & cook for a few seconds then slowly add the milk.

Add in the garlic powder; whisk well then add the cheeses.

Continue to stir the mixture until thick & bubbly, for a minute or two and then, add in the spinach leaves; stir well.

Broil until the top turn golden brown, for a couple of minutes.

Top with salsa, guacamole and queso; serve immediately & enjoy.

Nutrition: Calories: 459, Fat: 15 g, Carbs: 67 g, Protein: 15 g, Sodium: 1008 mg

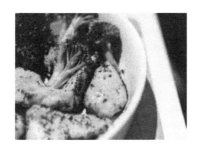 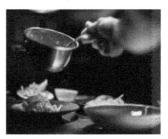

Awesome Blossom Petals

Preparation Time:15 minutes

Cooking Time: 15 minutes

Servings: 6

Ingredients:

For Seasoned Breading:

¼ teaspoon onion powder

2 ½ cups flour

½ teaspoon ground black pepper

2 teaspoons seasoned salt

½ teaspoon paprika

1 cup buttermilk

¼ teaspoon garlic powder

For Blossom Sauce:

1/8 teaspoon cayenne pepper

2 tablespoons ketchup

½ cup sour cream

1 ½ teaspoons prepared horseradish

½ teaspoon seasoned salt

Other **Ingredients:**

vegetable oil for frying

Directions:

For Blossom Sauce:

Combine the sour cream with ketchup, horseradish, cayenne pepper and seasoned salt in a small bowl; stir the ingredients well. Cover & let chill in a refrigerator until ready to serve.

For Onion:

Peel the onion.

Cut the stem of the onion off; place it on the cutting board, stem side down. Cut the onion horizontally and vertically into half then make two more diagonal cuts.

For Breading:

Add buttermilk in a large bowl.

Combine flour together with garlic powder, black pepper, paprika, onion powder and seasoned salt in a separate bowl. Using a large fork; give the ingredients a good stir until well mixed.

Put the onions first into the flour and then dip them into the buttermilk; then into the flour again. Let the onions to rest on the wire rack.

For Cooking:

Preheat oil until it reaches 350 F. Work in batches & add the onions into the hot oil (ensure that you don't overcrowd the onions); cook until turn golden brown, for 2 to 3 minutes.

Remove them from the hot oil & then place them on a wire rack to drain.

Serve hot & enjoy.

Nutrition: Calories: 158, Fat: 5 g, Carbs: 20 g, Protein:17 g

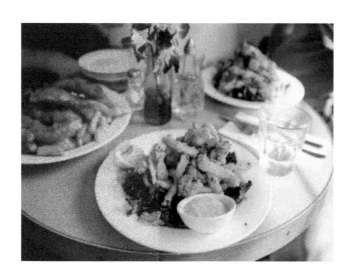

Chili's Buffalo wings

Preparation Time: 5 minutes

Cooking Time: 25 minutes

Servings: 2

Ingredients:

1 cup all-purpose flour

¼ cup hot sauce

1 cup 1% milk

¼ teaspoon paprika

5 cup vegetable oil

1 organic egg, large

2 chicken breast fillets; sliced into six pieces

1 tablespoon margarine

½ teaspoon black pepper

2 teaspoon salt

¼ teaspoon cayenne pepper

Directions:

In a large-sized mixing bowl; combine flour together with paprika, peppers and salt; mix well & set aside. Whisk the egg together with milk in a separate small-sized mixing bowl. Now, over moderate heat in a large, deep fryer; heat up 5 cups of the vegetable oil.

Dip each of your chicken pieces into the egg mixture and then into the breading blend. Continue to dip the pieces for one more time and ensure that all pieces are coated well. Set them on a plate to chill for 10 to 15 minutes.

Once done; carefully add the chicken pieces into the hot oil & fry until turn crispy & golden brown, for 4 to 5 minutes. In the meantime; combine the margarine with hot sauce in a separate mixing bowl & microwave until the margarine is melted, for 25 seconds.

When you are done with the chicken pieces; place them on a paper towel lined plate. Once done; place the chicken pieces into a plastic container & add the prepared sauce.

Close the container; shake well until the chicken is completely covered with the sauce. Serve immediately & enjoy.

Nutrition: Calories: 323, Fat: 34 g, Carbs: 7g, Protein:35 g, Sodium: 357 mg

Loaded Boneless Wings

Preparation Time: 30 minutes

Cooking Time: 50 minutes

Servings: 10

Ingredients:

For Veggie Queso Dip:

1 jalapeno pepper, finely chopped

½ yellow bell pepper, finely chopped

¼ teaspoon ground cumin

1 package American cheese, shredded (6 ounce)

½ red bell pepper, finely chopped

2 slices of Fontana cheese, shredded

½ teaspoon red pepper flakes

1 ball mozzarella cheese, shredded (4 ounce)

½ teaspoon olive oil

1/8 teaspoon each of garlic powder, ground black pepper, onion powder, ground nutmeg & salt

½ cup half-and-half

For Wings:

4 strips of bacon or to taste

1 package Buffalo-style boneless chicken breast halves, frozen (25.5 ounce)

½ pound cheddar cheese, shredded

3 green onions, thinly sliced

¼ pound Monterey Jack cheese, shredded

Directions:

Over medium heat in a large skillet; heat the olive oil until hot. Once done; add the yellow bell pepper together with red bell pepper & jalapeno pepper; stir well & cook for 2 to 3 minutes, until mostly tender, stirring constantly. Add the cumin; cook & stir for a minute more, until the peppers are nicely coated. Add half-&-half; let simmer until almost boiling. Decrease the heat to low and slowly stir in the mozzarella cheese, fontina cheese, American cheese, red pepper flakes, onion powder, garlic powder, nutmeg, black pepper and salt. Cook for 3 to 5 more minutes, until the cheeses are melted completely, stirring constantly.

Preheat oven to 400 F.

Place the frozen chicken breasts on a large-sized baking sheet & the bacon strips on a separate sheet.

Place both the pans in the preheated oven. Heat the chicken for 10 to 12 minutes, until thawed; remove from the oven. Continue to bake the bacon for 16 to 18 more minutes, until crispy. Leave the oven on; remove the bacon, place it on a paper towel to dry & then chop into pieces.

Place a cup of the prepared queso dip into the bottom of a large ovenproof dish or skillet. Arrange the chicken over the top & sprinkle with Monterey Jack cheese and Cheddar cheese.

Bake for 5 to 8 more minutes, until the cheeses have completely melted. Sprinkle with the chopped green onion and bacon pieces.

Nutrition: Calories: 377, Fat: 34 g, Carbs: 62 g, Protein: 21 g, Sodium: 647 mg

Classic Nachos

Preparation Time: 25 minutes

Cooking Time: 2 hours and 15 minutes

Servings: 5 persons

Ingredients:

2 tablespoon guacamole

1 boneless chicken breast, uncooked, cut in strips

A bag of tortilla chips, any of your choice

1 cup fresh lettuce, shredded

½ cup Monterey Jack cheese, shredded

1 package of fajita seasoning mix (1 ounces)

½ cup sharp cheddar cheese, shredded

1 jalapeño, sliced

½ cup your choice salsa

1 Vidalia onion, sliced

2 tablespoon low-fat sour cream

1 bell pepper, sliced

Directions:

Over moderate heat in a large skillet; sauté the chicken with onion, fajita seasoning & peppers. When done; drain the prepared fajita mixture & set aside until ready to use.

Now, spread the tortillas out on your ovenproof platter in a large circle. Once done; start layering them with chicken, peppers and onions. Add the cheeses followed by the jalapenos. Place the platter into the oven & bake until the cheese is completely melted, for 5 to 10 minutes, at 350

F. Once done; pull out the platter & add the shredded lettuce in the center of chip circle. Top the lettuce with sour cream, salsa & guacamole. Serve immediately & enjoy.

Nutrition: Calories: 345, Fat: 14 g, Carbs: 34 g, Protein:54 g, Sodium: 1435 mg

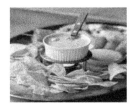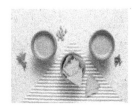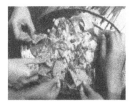

Fried Pickles

Preparation Time: 5 minutes

Cooking Time: 10 minutes

Servings: 4

Ingredients:

2 cup pickle chips

¼ teaspoon cayenne pepper

1 teaspoon sugar

½ teaspoon pepper

2 cup flour

Oil, for frying

1 teaspoon salt

Directions:

Over moderate heat in a deep pan; heat the oil until hot. Now, in a large bowl; combine the flour together with cayenne, sugar, pepper, and salt; continue to whisk until combined well.

Drain the pickle chips & then toss them into the prepared flour mixture. Once done, work in batches and fry them (ensure that you don't overcrowd the pan). Once the pickles starts to float to the surface, immediately remove them from the hot oil. Place them on paper towels to drain; serve with the horseradish or ranch dressing and enjoy.

Nutrition: Calories: 266, Fat: 20 g, Carbs: 34 g, Protein: 23 g, Sodium: 624 mg

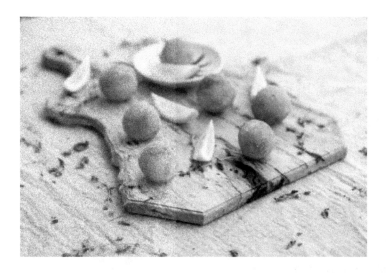

Crispy Cheddar Bites

Preparation Time: 15 minutes

Cooking Time: 20 minutes

Servings: 4

Ingredients:

1 cup all-purpose flour

½ cup softened butter, at room temperature (1 stick)

1 cup sharp cheddar cheese, shredded, slightly packed

1/8 teaspoon cayenne pepper

1 cup crispy rice cereal

¼ teaspoon salt

Directions:

Preheat oven to 375 F. Lightly coat two rimmed baking sheets with the cooking spray.

Using a wooden spoon; combine the entire ingredients together in a large bowl; continue to mix until thoroughly mixed. Make 1" balls from the prepared mixture & arrange them on coated baking sheets. Slightly flatten the balls using the bottom of a drinking glass or the palm of your hand.

Bake in the preheated oven until the edges turn golden brown, for 10 to 12 minutes. Serve warm & enjoy.

Nutrition: Calories: 366, Fat: 25 g, Carbs: 45 g, Protein:42 g, Sodium: 428 mg

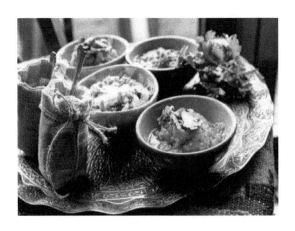

Texas Chili Fries

Preparation Time: 10 minutes

Cooking Time: 20 minutes

Servings: 4

Ingredients:

1 package of bacon

1 bag cheese blend, shredded

Ranch salad dressing

1 bag steak fries, frozen

1 jar jalapeno peppers

Directions:

Evenly spread the fries over a large-sized cookie sheet & bake as per the directions mentioned on the package.

Line strips of bacon on a separate cookie sheet & bake until crispy.

When the bacon and fries are done; remove them from the oven.

Add a thick layer of jalapenos and cheese; crumble the bacon over the fries.

Bake in the oven again until the cheese is completely melted.

Serve hot with some Ranch salad dressing on side and enjoy.

Nutrition: Calories: 537, Fat: 17 g, Carbs: 56 g, Protein: 36 g, Sodium: 683 mg

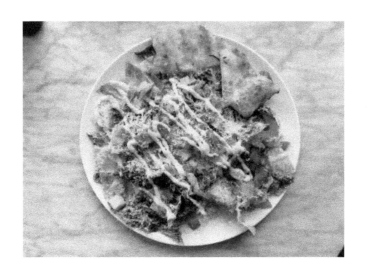

Chili's Salad

Preparation Time: 25 minutes

Cooking Time: 15 minutes

Servings: 4

Ingredients:

For Pico De Gallo:

2 teaspoon seeded jalapeno peppers, finely diced

½ cup red onion finely minced

2 medium tomatoes diced very small

2 teaspoon cilantro, fresh & finely minced

For Salad:

4 chicken breasts skinless, boneless

5 ounces bag half-and-half spring mix with baby spinach

½ cup red cabbage chopped

6.5 ounces bag butter bliss lettuce or romaine or iceberg lettuce

¾ cup craisins

1 cup fresh pineapple chunked

¼ cup teriyaki sauce

14 ounces can mandarin orange segments drained

Tortilla strips

¼ cup water

For Honey-Lime Dressing:

1 cup vanilla Greek yogurt

¼ cup Dijon mustard

1 tablespoon lime juice, freshly squeezed

3 tablespoon apple cider vinegar

1 cup honey

2 tablespoon sesame oil

½ to 1 teaspoon lime zest grated

Directions:

For Pico De Gallo:

Combine the ingredients for Pico de Gallo together in a small bowl & let chill in a refrigerator until ready to use.

For Salad:

1. Mix the teriyaki sauce with water.

Place the chicken pieces in a large-sized plastic bag or plastic bowl.

Add in the prepared teriyaki mixture & let marinate for an hour or two in the refrigerator.

Layer the lettuce & spring mix in large serving bowl.

Add craisins and cabbage; toss well.

Refrigerate until all ingredients are ready.

After chicken has marinated; lightly coat your grill with the cooking spray and heat it over moderate heat.

Remove the chicken pieces from marinade; shaking off any excess.

Add to the hot grill & cook until the chicken is cooked through, for 5 to 10 minutes on each side.

Slice chicken down into cubes or thin strips. Set aside on the serving plate to serve.

For Honey-Lime Dressing:

Combine the entire salad dressing ingredients in a blender; blend on high until blended well.

Refrigerate until ready to serve.

To Assemble the Salad:

Remove the salad to four individual large serving plates.

Place approximately ¼ cup of the mandarin orange segments & pineapple over each salad.

Sprinkle with the chicken.

Top with a spoonful or two of Pico de Gallo or to taste.

Drizzle with salad dressing; give the ingredients a good stir until mixed well.

Garnish with the tortilla strips. Serve immediately & enjoy.

Nutrition: Calories: 535, Fat: 33 g, Carbs: 24 g, Protein: 51 g, Sodium: 635 mg

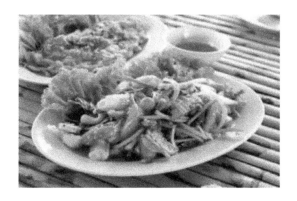

Raspberry Lemonade

Preparation Time: 2 minutes

Cooking Time: 3 minutes

Servings: 8

Ingredients:

1 cup water

1 cup sugar

1 cup freshly squeezed lemon juice

1 ½ cups fresh or frozen raspberries

Extra sugar for the rim of your glass

Directions:

In a small saucepan, heat the water and sugar until the sugar completely dissolves.

Meanwhile, purée the raspberries in a blender. Add the contents of the saucepan and the cup of lemon juice. (If it's too thick you can add extra water.)

Wet the rim of your glass and dip it into a bit of sugar to coat the rim before pouring the lemonade into the glass.

Nutrition: Calories: 234, Fat: 56. 2 g, Carbs: 23. 8 g, Protein: 23. 5 g, Sodium: 1324 mg

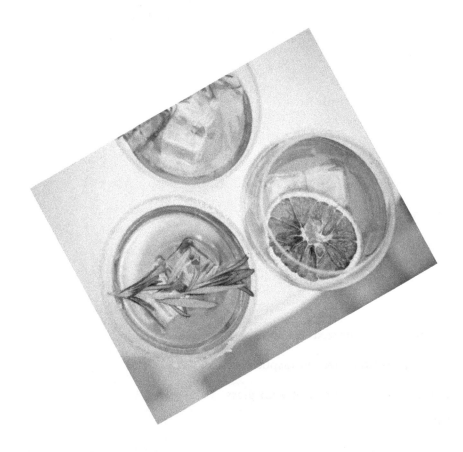

Lunch (Chicken)

Alice Springs Chicken from Outback

Preparation Time: 5 minutes

Cooking Time: 2 hours and 30 minutes

Servings: 4

Ingredients:

Sauce:

½ cup Dijon mustard

½ cup honey

¼ cup mayonnaise

1 teaspoon fresh lemon juice

Chicken preparation:

4 chicken breast, boneless and skinless

2 tablespoons butter

1 tablespoon olive oil

8 ounces fresh mushrooms, sliced

4 slices bacon, cooked and cut into 2-inch pieces

2 ½ cups Monterrey Jack cheese, shredded

Parsley for serving (optional)

Directions:

Preheat oven to 400 °F.

Mix together ingredients for the sauce in a bowl.

Put chicken in a Ziploc bag, then add sauce into bag until only ¼ cup is left. Keep remaining sauce in a container, cover, and refrigerate. Make sure to seal Ziploc bag tightly and shake gently until chicken is coated with sauce Keep in refrigerator for at least 2 hours.

Melt butter in a pan over medium heat. Toss in mushrooms and cook for 5 minutes or until brown. Remove from pan and place on a plate.

In an oven-safe pan, heat oil. Place marinated chicken flat in pan and cook for 5 minutes on each side or until both sides turn golden brown.

Nutrition: Calories: 888, Fat: 56 g, Carbs: 41 g, Protein: 59 g, Sodium: 1043 mg

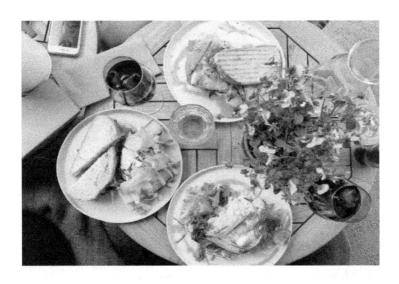

Panda Express' Orange Chicken

Preparation Time: 15 minutes

Cooking Time: 30 minutes

Servings: 6

Ingredients:

Orange sauce:

1½ tablespoon soy sauce

1½ tablespoon water

5 tablespoons sugar

5 tablespoons white vinegar

3 tablespoons orange zest

Chicken preparation:

1 egg - 1½ teaspoon salt

White pepper, to taste

5 tablespoons grapeseed oil, divided

½ cup + 1 tablespoon cornstarch

¼ cup flour

¼ cup cold water

2 pounds chicken breast, boneless and skinless, chopped

1 teaspoon fresh ginger, grated

1 teaspoon garlic, finely chopped

½ teaspoon hot red chili pepper, ground

¼ cup green onion, sliced 1 tablespoon rice wine

½ teaspoon sesame oil

White rice and steamed broccoli for serving

Directions:

Mix together ingredients for the orange sauce in a bowl. Reserve for later.

Add egg, salt, pepper, and 1 tablespoon oil to a separate bowl. Mix well.

In another bowl, combine ½ cup cornstarch and flour. Mix until fully blended.

Add remaining cornstarch and cold water in a different bowl. Blend until cornstarch is completely dissolved.

Heat 3 tablespoons oil in a large deep skillet or wok over high heat.

Coat chicken pieces in egg mixture. Let excess drip off. Then, coat in cornstarch mixture. Cook for at least 3 minutes or until both sides are golden brown and chicken is cooked through. Arrange on a plate lined with paper towels to drain excess oil.

In a clean large deep skillet, or wok heat remaining oil on high heat. Lightly sauté ginger and garlic for 30 seconds or until aromatic. Toss in peppers and green onions. Stir-fry vegetables for 1-3 minutes, then pour in rice wine. Mix well before adding orange sauce. Bring to a boil. Mix in cooked chicken pieces, then add cornstarch mixture. Simmer until mixture is thick, then mix in sesame oil.

Transfer onto a plate and serve with white rice and steamed broccoli.

Nutrition: Calories: 305, Fat: 5 g, Carbs: 27 g, Protein: 34 g, Sodium: 1024 mg

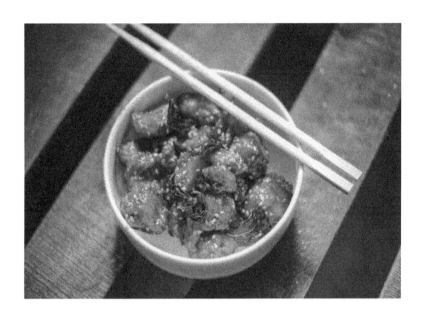

Chili's Boneless Buffalo Wings

Preparation Time: 30 minutes

Cooking Time: 15 minutes

Servings: 2

Ingredients:

1 cup flour

2 teaspoons salt

½ teaspoon black pepper, ground

¼ teaspoon cayenne pepper, ground

1 egg

1 cup milk

5 cups vegetable oil

2 chicken breasts, boneless and skinless, cut into 6 pieces

¼ cup hot sauce

1 tablespoon margarine

1 blue cheese salad dressing

1 stalk celery, cut into sticks

Directions:

In a bowl, mix together flour, salt, peppers, and paprika.

Add egg and milk to a separate bowl and mix well.

Preheat 5 cups oil in a deep-fryer to 375 °F.

Coat chicken pieces into egg mixture. Allow excess to drip off, then coat with flour mixture. Repeat twice for a double coat.

Transfer breaded chicken onto a plate and refrigerate for about 15 minutes.

Deep-fry each for about 5 minutes or until brown and transfer onto a paper towel-lined plate.

Meanwhile, mix hot sauce and margarine in a bowl. Then, heat in the microwave for about 20 seconds or until melted. Mix well until fully blended.

Place chicken pieces in a large Ziploc bag and add sauce. Seal bag tightly. Using your hands, mix chicken and sauce together until well-coated.

Serve chicken pieces on a plate with blue cheese dressing and celery sticks on the side.

Nutrition: Calories: 398, Fat: 13 g, Carbs: 55 g, Protein: 14 g, Sodium: 3234 mg

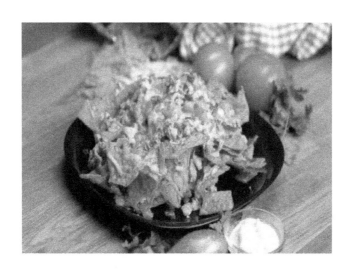

Boston Market's Rotisserie Chicken Copycat

Preparation Time: 24 hours

Cooking Time: 1 hour

Servings: 4

Ingredients:

¼ cup apple cider vinegar

½ cup canola oil

2 tablespoons brown sugar

4 fresh garlic cloves, finely chopped

1 whole roasting chicken

Directions:

Combine vinegar, oil, sugar, and garlic in a bowl. Add chicken and spoon mixture on top to coat well. Refrigerate overnight, making sure to turn chicken over to soak opposite side

Remove chicken from refrigerator. Set aside for at least 20 minutes.

Bake at 350°F for about 45-50 minutes or until the temperature reads 165°F on an instant meat thermometer inserted in thickest part of the thigh without touching any bones.

Serve.

Nutrition: Calories: 433, Fat: 39 g, Carbs: 8 g, Protein: 13 g, Sodium: 53 mg

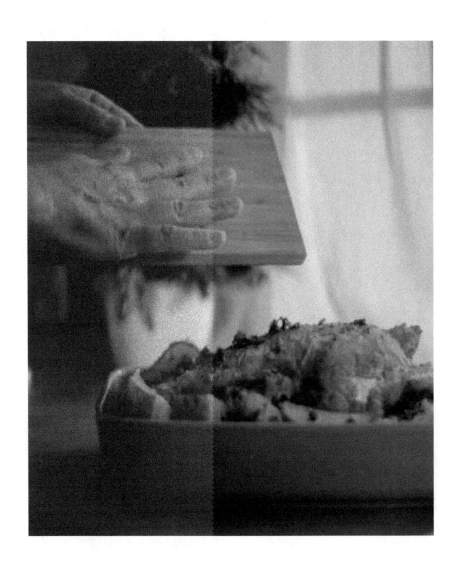

Cracker Barrel Chicken and Dumplings

Preparation Time: 1 hour

Cooking Time: 2 hours

Servings: 6

Ingredients:

1 whole chicken

2 quarts water

2 teaspoons salt

½ teaspoon pepper

2 cups all-purpose flour

½ teaspoon baking soda

½ teaspoon salt

3 tablespoons shortening

¾ cup buttermilk

Directions:

In a heavy bottomed pot, boil chicken in water mixed with salt. Cover, then lower heat. Simmer for about 1 hour or until tender enough that the meat almost falls off the bone.

Using a slotted spoon, transfer chicken to a plate and cool. Then, remove bones and chop into small pieces.

In same pot, add broth and bring to a boil Add pepper.

In a bowl, mix flour, baking soda, and salt. Fold in shortening. Pour in buttermilk and mix everything until incorporated.

Knead dough 4 to 5 times. Pinch off about ½ inche size balls of dough and to the boiling broth. Reduce heat to medium-low. Simmer for about 8 to 10 minutes while stirring every now and then.

Add chicken to pot and stir.

Serve immediately.

Nutrition: Calories: 711, Fat: 41 g, Saturated fat: 12 g, Carbs: 33 g, Sugar: 2 g, Fibers: 1 g, Protein: 48 g, Sodium: 1276 mg

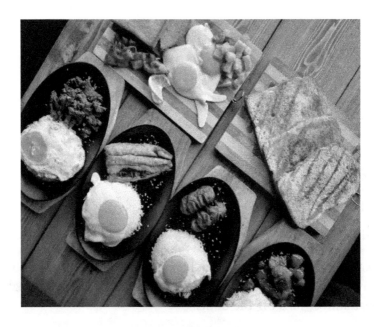

Chipotle's Chicken

Preparation Time: 10 minutes

Cooking Time: 20 minutes

Marinate Time: 24 hours

Servings: 8

Ingredients:

2 ½ pound organic boneless and skinless chicken breasts or thighs

Olive oil or cooking spray

Marinade

7 oz. chipotle peppers in adobo sauce

2 tablespoons olive oil

6 garlic cloves, peeled

1 teaspoon black pepper

2 teaspoons salt

½ teaspoon cumin

½ teaspoon dry oregano

Directions:

Pour all the marinade ingredients in a food processor or blender and blend until you get a smooth paste.

Pound the chicken until it has a thickness between ½ to ¾ inch. Place chicken into an airtight container or re-sealable plastic bag such as a Ziploc. Pour the marinade over the chicken and stir until well coated. Place the chicken in the refrigerator and let marinate overnight or up to 24 hours.

Pour the blended mixture into the container and marinate the chicken for at least 8 hours.

Cook the chicken over medium to high heat on an oiled and preheated grill for 3 to 5 minutes per side. The internal temperature of the chicken should be 165°F before you remove it from the heat. You can also cook it in heavy bottomed skillet over medium heat with a little olive oil.

Let rest before serving. If desired, cut into cubes to add to salads, tacos or quesadillas or serve as is.

Nutrition: Calories: 293, Fat: 18.7 g, Carbs: 5.8 g, Protein: 24.9 g, Sodium: 526 mg

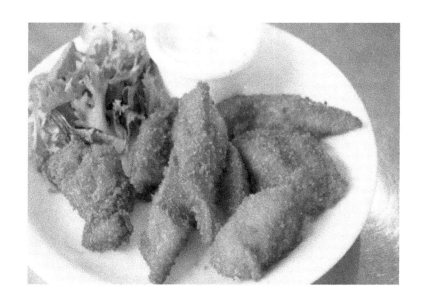

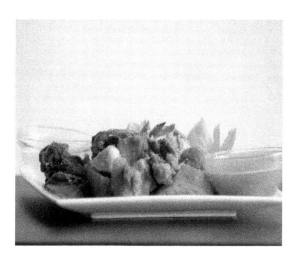

Popeye's Fried Chicken

Preparation Time: 20 minutes

Cooking Time: 45 minutes

Servings: 8

Ingredients:

Breading:

3 cups self-rising flour

1 cup corn starch

3 tablespoons seasoning salt

2 tablespoons paprika

1 teaspoon baking soda

1 package (0.7 ounce) dry Italian-style salad dressing mix

1 package (1 ounce) dry onion soup mix

1 (1 ½ ounces) packet dry spaghetti sauce spices and seasoning mix

3 tablespoons white sugar

Batter/Coating:

3 cups cornflakes cereal, crushed

2 eggs, beaten

¼ cup cold water

Chicken:

2 cups oil for frying

1 (4-pound) whole chicken, cut into pieces

Directions:

Mix all of the breading ingredients together in a deep bowl.

Place the crushed cereal in another bowl.

In another bowl, beat the eggs and cold water together.

Heat the oil to 350°F and preheat the oven to 350°F.

Dip the chicken into the breading mixture, the egg mixture, the crushed cereal, and then the breading mixture again.

Immediately place the breaded chicken into the heated oil and cook on each side for 3 to 4 minutes.

Place the chicken in a 9×13 baking pan skin-side up. Cover the baking pan with foil, leaving a small opening.

Bake the chicken for 45 minutes.

After 45 minutes, remove the foil and continue baking for another 5 minutes.

Remove the baking pan from the oven and serve.

Nutrition: Calories: 733, Fat: 26.8 g, Carbs: 76.3 g, Protein: 44.3 g, Sodium: 3140 mg

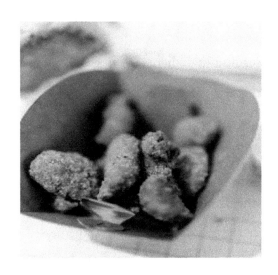

McDonald's Chicken Nuggets

Preparation Time: 45 minutes

Cooking Time: 45 minutes

Servings: 4

Ingredients:

Chicken:

1 pound chicken tenderloins, boneless and thawed

Brine:

4 cups water, cold

2 teaspoons fine sea salt

Breading:

⅓ + ½ cup all-purpose flour, sifted

All-purpose flour, sifted

½ cup corn starch

1½ tablespoons seasoned salt

1 tablespoon fine corn flour

1½ teaspoons dry milk powder, non-fat

1 teaspoon granulated sugar

½ teaspoon ginger, ground

¼ teaspoon mustard, ground

¼ teaspoon black pepper, fine

¼ teaspoon white pepper, fine

⅛ teaspoon allspice, ground

⅛ teaspoon cloves, ground

⅛ teaspoon paprika, ground

⅛ teaspoon turmeric, ground

1 pinch cinnamon, ground

1 pinch cayenne pepper

Batter:

2 eggs, beaten

½ cup water, cold

2 tablespoons corn starch

2 tablespoons all-purpose flour

¼ teaspoon sea salt, fine

¼ teaspoon sesame oil

¼ teaspoon soy sauce

¼ teaspoon granulated sugar

For Deep Frying:

Vegetable oil, 3 parts

Vegetable shortening, 1 part

Directions:

Pound the chicken until it is only ½ inch thick.

Mix the brine ingredients.

Cut the chicken into small, chicken-nugget-sized pieces and place them in the brine. Leave it in the refrigerator for 2 hours.

When the chicken is almost done soaking, whisk together all the batter ingredients. Also mix together all the breading ingredients.

Remove the chicken from the refrigerator and evenly coat each piece with the batter.

Evenly coat each battered piece with the breading.

Slowly heat the deep-frying ingredients to 350°F.

Deep fry each nugget and then transfer to a plate with a paper towel to drain the oil.

Transfer to a different plate and serve.

Note: The nuggets can be battered up and breaded in advance and stored in an airtight container if you want to fry them later

Nutrition: Calories: 370.5, Fat: 5 g, Carbs: 44.9 g, Protein: 33.2 g, Sodium: 1457.4 mg

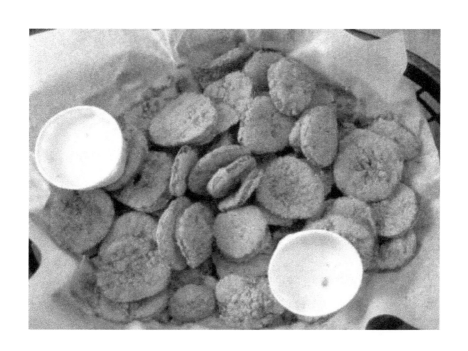

Ruby Tuesday's Sonora Chicken Pasta

Preparation Time: 25 minutes

Cooking Time: 20 minutes

Servings: 4

Ingredients:

Cheese Mixture

1 pound processed cheese like Velveeta

½ cup heavy cream

2 teaspoons olive oil

2 tablespoons red chili peppers, minced

2 tablespoons green chili peppers, minced

2 tablespoons onions, minced

½ garlic clove, minced

2 tablespoons water

¼ teaspoon salt

2 teaspoons sugar

½ tablespoon vinegar

¼ teaspoon cumin

Beans:

1 can 15-ounce can black beans, with the water

2 tablespoons green chili peppers, minced

2 tablespoons onions, minced

½ garlic clove, minced

¼ teaspoon salt

1 dash paprika

Seasoning and Chicken:

Vegetable oil

½ teaspoon salt

1 dash dried thyme

1 dash dried summer savory

4 chicken breast halves, boneless, skinless

Pasta:

1 box (16 ounces) penne pasta

4 quarts water

1 tablespoon butter

Garnish:

Green onion, chopped

Tomatoes, diced

Directions:

Preheat your grill.

Mix the Velveeta and the cream over heat until smooth.

In another pan, heat the olive oil and sauté the peppers, onions, and garlic clove.

After 2 minutes, add the water and bring to a simmer for another 2 minutes.

Add the sautéed vegetables to the cheese and continue simmering over low heat. Add in the salt, the sugar, the vinegar, and the cumin, and leave the entire mixture over low heat. Make sure to stir.

In another saucepan, bring the beans, peppers, onions, garlic, salt, and paprika to a boil over medium heat.

When the bean mixture starts boiling, reduce the heat to low and keep it simmering.

Mix all the seasoning ingredients and then rub the seasoning all over the chicken.

Cook the chicken in oil thoroughly, for 5 minutes on each side, and then slice the chicken pieces into ½-inch slices.

Boil the pasta in the water. When it is cooked, drain the pasta and mix in the butter while the noodles are still hot.

Assemble the dish by covering the pasta in sauce, placing the bean mixture over it, and then adding the chicken. Garnish the dish by topping everything with the tomatoes and green onions.

Nutrition: Calories: 966, Fat: 18 g, Carbs: 34 g, Protein: 0 g, Sodium: 0 g

Olive Garden's Chicken Marsala

Preparation Time: 10 minutes

Cooking Time: 40 minutes

Servings: 6

Ingredients:

2 tablespoons olive oil

2 tablespoons butter

4 boneless skinless chicken breasts

1 ½ cups sliced mushrooms

1 small clove garlic, thinly sliced

Flour for dredging

Sea salt and freshly ground black pepper

1 ½ cups chicken stock

1 ½ cups Marsala wine

1 tablespoon lemon juice

1 teaspoon Dijon mustard

Directions:

Chicken scaloppini

Pound out the chicken with a mallet or rolling pin to about ½ inch thick

In a large skillet, heat the olive oil and 1 tablespoon of the butter over medium-high heat. When the oil is hot, dredge the chicken in flour. Season with salt and pepper on both sides. Dredge only as many as will fit in the skillet. Don't overcrowd the pan.

Cook chicken in batches, about 1 to 2 minutes on each side or until cooked through. Remove from skillet, and place on an oven-proof platter. Keep warm, in oven, while remaining chicken is cooked.

Marsala sauce

In the same skillet, add 1 tablespoon of olive oil. On medium-high heat, sauté mushrooms and garlic until softened. Remove the mushrooms from the pan and set aside.

Add the chicken stock and loosen any remaining bits in the pan. On high heat, let reduce by half, about 6-8 minutes. Add Marsala wine and lemon juice and in the same manner reduce by half, about 6–8 minutes. Add the mushroom back in the saucepan, and stir in the Dijon mustard. Warm for 1 minute on medium-low heat. Remove from heat, stir in the remaining butter to make the sauce silkier.

To serve, pour sauce over chicken, and serve immediately.

Nutrition: Calories: 950, Fat: 58 g, Carbs: 71 g, Protein: 66 g, Sodium: 1910 mg

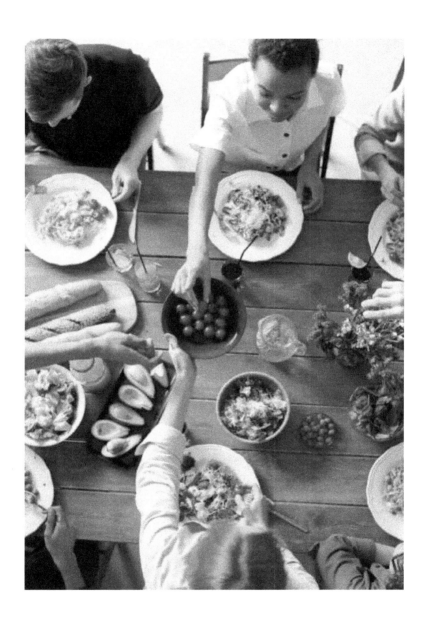

Chili's Crispy Honey-Chipotle Chicken Crispers

Preparation Time: 15 minutes

Cooking Time: 30 minutes

Servings: 4

Ingredients:

Chicken: 12 chicken tenderloins

Some shortening or 6 cups vegetable oil for frying

Honey-Chipotle Sauce:

⅔ cup honey

¼ cup water

¼ cup ketchup

1 tablespoon white vinegar

2 teaspoons chipotle chili pepper, ground or powdered

½ teaspoon salt

Batter:

1 egg, beaten

½ cup whole milk

½ cup chicken broth

1½ teaspoons salt

¼ teaspoon black pepper

¼ teaspoon paprika

¼ teaspoon garlic powder

¾ cup all-purpose flour

Breading:

1½ cups all-purpose flour

1½ teaspoons salt

¾ teaspoon paprika

½ teaspoon black pepper

½ teaspoon garlic powder

Garnish:

French fries

Corn on the cub

Ranch dipping sauce

Directions:

Mix together all the chipotle sauce ingredients in a saucepan and bring to a boil over medium heat. When the sauce starts boiling, reduce it to a simmer and leave it for another two minutes before removing from heat.

Preheat the oil to 350°F. While you are waiting for your oil to heat, whisk all the batter ingredients (except the flour) together for 30 seconds, or until thoroughly mixed. When everything is mixed, add in the flour and mix again.

Add all the breading ingredients to another bowl.

Place the batter and breading bowls beside each other to make your coating station. The oil should be hot enough now.

Dip the chicken into the batter, let the excess batter drip off, and then dip it in the breading to coat.

Place the breaded chicken on a plate and start frying, two at a time at most. Leave each chicken piece in the oil for at least 4 minutes.

Prepare a plate by covering it with paper towels.

When the chicken is done cooking, transfer it to the paper towels to let the oil drain off.

Let the fried chicken cool, and then transfer it to a deep bowl. Add in the sauce and toss everything together. Make sure you cover the chicken in sauce.

Transfer to a plate and serve with sides of French fries, corn on the cub, and ranch dipping sauce.

Nutrition: Calories: 492, Fat: 3.3 g, Carbs: 107.2 g, Protein: 11.2 g, Sodium: 2331.5 mg

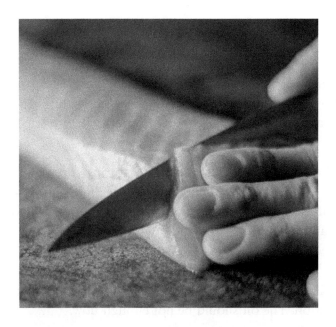

Lunch (Fish)

Applebee's Honey Grilled Salmon

Preparation Time: 10 minutes

Cooking Time: 30 minutes

Servings: 4

Ingredients:

Honey Pepper Sauce:

¾ cup honey

⅓ cup soy sauce

¼ cup dark brown sugar, packed

¼ cup pineapple juice

2 tablespoons fresh lemon juice

2 tablespoons white distilled vinegar

2 teaspoons olive oil

1 teaspoon black pepper, ground

½ teaspoon cayenne pepper

½ teaspoon paprika

¼ teaspoon garlic powder

Fish:

4 salmon fillets, 8 ounces each, skinned

Directions:

Cook all of the sauce ingredients over medium to low heat until boiling. Once the mixture boils, lower the heat a little and allow it to simmer for another 15 minutes.

Rub the salmon with vegetable oil, salt, and pepper, and grill for 4 to 7 minutes on each side.

Serve with the honey pepper sauce.

Nutrition: Calories: 579.6, Fat: 12.3 g, Carbs: 70.5 g, Protein: 49 g, Sodium: 1515.1 mg

Red Lobster's Maple-Glazed Salmon and Shrimp

Preparation Time: 10 minutes

Cooking Time: 20 minutes

Servings: 4

Ingredients:

⅔ cup maple syrup

½ cup water

2 tablespoons dried cherries, minced

1 tablespoon sugar

2 teaspoons soy sauce

1½ teaspoons lemon juice

24 pieces fresh medium shrimp, peeled

24 ounces salmon fillets

Directions:

To get started:

a) Skewer the shrimp on 4 skewers (i.e. 6 shrimp each);

b) Season the shrimp with salt and pepper; and

c) Season the salmon with salt and pepper.

Combine the maple syrup, water, cherries, sugar soy sauce and lemon juice and bring to a boil over medium heat. Reduce the heat and allow the mixture to simmer for another 8 to 10 minutes.

Grill the shrimp over high heat for 1 to 2 minutes per side. When you're done with the shrimp, grill the salmon over high heat for 3 to 4 minutes per side.

Arrange the shrimp and salmon on a plate and serve with the maple sauce.

Nutrition: Calories: 364.7, Fat: 7.4 g, Carbs: 38.7 g, Protein: 34.8 g, Sodium: 301.1 mg

Chili's Garlic and Lime Shrimp

Preparation Time: 5 minutes

Cooking Time: 20 minutes

Servings: 4

Ingredients:

Shrimp:

2 tablespoons butter

1 clove garlic, chopped

32 fresh medium shrimp, peeled

1 lime, halved

Seasoning:

¾ teaspoon salt

¼ teaspoon ground black pepper

¼ teaspoon cayenne pepper

¼ teaspoon dried parsley flakes

¼ teaspoon garlic powder

¼ teaspoon paprika

⅛ teaspoon dried thyme

⅛ teaspoon onion powder

Directions:

Stir all the seasoning ingredients together to make the seasoning mix.

Sauté the garlic in the butter over medium heat for a few seconds before adding the shrimp to the pan. Squeeze the lime over the shrimp and continue to sauté it.

Stir in the seasoning mix, and continue sautéing the mixture for another 5 to 8 minutes.

Transfer to a plate and serve with thin lime wedges.

Nutrition: Calories: 89.1, Fat: 6.3 g, Carbs: 2.9 g, Protein: 6 g, Sodium: 725.4 mg

Red Lobster's Nantucket Baked Cod

Preparation Time: 10 minutes

Cooking Time: 30 minutes

Servings: 4

Ingredients:

Fish:

4 fresh cod fish fillets, about 1 ½ pounds in total

1 tablespoon butter, melted

½ lemon, juiced

2 small tomatoes, sliced

2 tablespoons grated parmesan cheese

Spice Blend:

¼ teaspoon salt

¼ teaspoon paprika

1 dash black pepper

1 dash cayenne pepper

Directions:

To get started:

a)   Preheat the oven to 450°F; and

b)   Prepare a 9×13 baking pan.

Place all the ingredients for the spice blend in a bowl and mix thoroughly.

Place the cod filets in the baking pan and brush with the tops with the butter.

Sprinkle the lemon juice and spice blend over the filets until you have finished all the spice blend.

Place 2 to 3 tomato slices on top of the spices for each fish.

Cover each slice of tomato with parmesan cheese.

Bake the fish for 8 minutes, then broil it on high for another 6 to 8 minutes.

Transfer the fish to a serving dish and serve with rice.

Nutrition: Calories: 187.9, Fat: 4.9 g, Carbs: 2.8 g, Protein: 31.9 g, Sodium: 303.6 mg

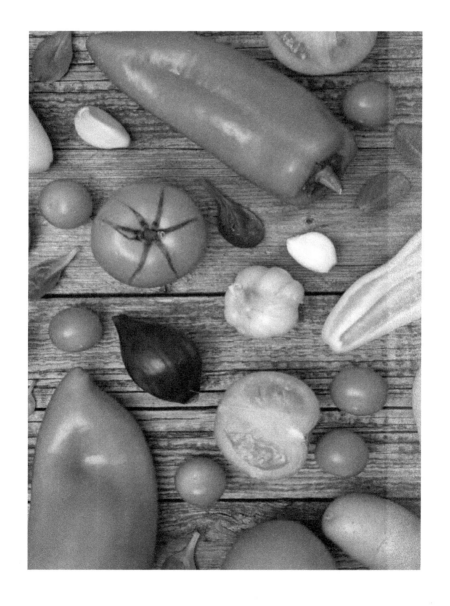

Chili's Crunchy Fried Shrimp

Preparation Time: 10 minutes

Cooking Time: 1 minute

Servings: 8

Ingredients:

2 pounds large shrimp, peeled

Crisco shortening, melted

Corn flake crumbs

Batter:

⅔ cup flour

1⅓ cups cornstarch

½ teaspoon salt

½ teaspoon baking powder

6 egg whites

⅔ cup water

4 tablespoons vegetable oil

Directions:

Mix the batter ingredients together and set aside.

In a separate container, pour out the cornflake crumbs.

Preheat the oil over medium heat.

Coat each shrimp with a generous amount of batter and then roll it in the crumbs.

Deep fry the shrimp until golden brown.

Place the shrimp on oil absorbent paper or paper towels.

Serve with cocktail or tartar sauce.

Nutrition: Calories: 272.9, Fat: 8.1 g, Carbs: 28.7 g, Protein: 19.3 g, Sodium: 854.2 mg

Applebee's Garlic and Peppercorn Fried Shrimp

Preparation Time:5 minutes

Cooking Time: 30 minutes

Servings: 4

Ingredients:

Shrimp:

1 pound shrimp, peeled, deveined, and tail removed

Vegetable oil, as needed

Flour Mixture:

½ cup wheat flour

¼ teaspoon salt

1 teaspoon ground black pepper

1 teaspoon granulated garlic

½ teaspoon paprika

1 teaspoon granulated sugar

Eggs:

2 eggs, beaten

Breading:

1 cup breadcrumbs

1 teaspoon ground black pepper

Directions:

Heat 3 inches of oil to 350°F.

Place the ingredients for the flour mixture in a bowl and mix. In separate bowls, beat the eggs and mix the breading ingredients together.

Dip the eggs in the flour mixture, then the eggs, then the breading.

After dipping, place the shrimp directly into the heated oil and cook for 2 to 3 minutes.

Place the cooked shrimp on a serving plate and serve with ketchup or tartar sauce.

Nutrition: Calories: 284.4, Fat: 5.4 g, Carbs: 34 g, Protein: 24.4 g , Sodium: 1021.5 mg

Cheesecake Factory's Bang Bang Chicken and Shrimp

Preparation Time: 10 minutes

Cooking Time: 50 minutes

Servings: 4

Ingredients:

Curry Sauce:

2 teaspoons chili oil

¼ cup onion

2 tablespoons garlic cloves, minced

2 teaspoons ginger

1 cup chicken broth

½ teaspoon cumin, ground

½ teaspoon coriander, ground

½ teaspoon paprika

¼ teaspoon salt

¼ teaspoon black pepper, ground

¼ teaspoon mace, ground

¼ teaspoon turmeric

3 cups coconut milk

2 medium carrots, julienned

1 small zucchini, julienned

½ cup peas, frozen

Peanut Sauce:

¼ cup creamy peanut butter

2 tablespoons water

4 teaspoons sugar

1 tablespoon soy sauce

1 teaspoon rice vinegar

1 teaspoon lime juice

½ teaspoon chili oil

Protein:

2 chicken breast fillets, cut into bite-sized pieces

16 large shrimp, raw, shelled

¼ cup cornstarch

½ cup vegetable oil

Final Dish:

1½ cups flaked coconut

4 cups white rice, cooked

½ teaspoon dried parsley, crumbled

2 tablespoons peanuts, finely chopped

2 green onions, julienned

Directions:

Sauté the onion, garlic, and ginger in heated chili oil for 30 seconds before adding in the broth.

Cook the mixture for another 30 seconds and then add in the cumin, coriander, paprika, salt, pepper, mace and turmeric.

Stir everything together and bring to a simmer. Keep the mixture at a simmer for 5 minutes and then add the coconut milk.

After adding the coconut milk, bring the mixture to a boil for 20 seconds.

Reduce the heat and then allow the mixture to simmer for 20 minutes before adding the carrots, zucchini, and peas.

Simmer the entire mixture for another 20 minutes and set the curry sauce aside. While waiting for the mixture to thicken, preheat the oven to 300°F.

Next, prepare the peanut sauce by mixing all of the ingredients together over medium heat.

When the peanut sauce starts to bubble, cover the pot, remove from heat, and set aside.

Spread the flaked coconut on a baking pan and bake for 30 minutes to toast. Swirl the flakes every 10 minutes, making sure they do not burn.

Pour the cornstarch in a bowl. Place the prepared chicken and shrimp into the bowl and cover entirely.

Sauté the chicken in the vegetable oil until it is cooked. Add the shrimp to the chicken and continue cooking.

Transfer the protein to a plate and set aside.

Arrange the dish as follows:

a)   Place some rice in the center of a plate;

b)   Place the chicken and shrimp around the rice;

c)   Pour the curry sauce over the chicken and the shrimp;

d)   Drizzle the peanut sauce over everything—especially the rice;

e)   Sprinkle some parsley and peanuts over the top of the rice, then top with the onions; then

f)   Sprinkle the toasted coconut flakes over the dish.

Serve and enjoy.

Nutrition: Calories: 1211, Fat: 84.2 g, Carbs: 101 g, Protein: 30 g, Sodium: 1940 mg

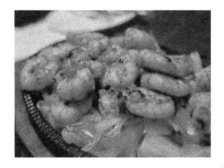

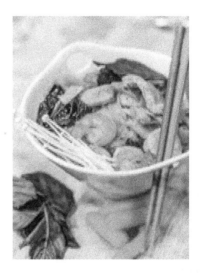

Disney World's Fulton's Crab House's Dungeness Crab Cakes

Preparation Time: 15 minutes

Cooking Time: 40 minutes

Servings: 4

Ingredients:

2½ pounds Dungeness crabmeat

1⅛ cups unsalted soda crackers, crushed

⅛ cup Dijon mustard

½ teaspoon Old Bay Seasoning

⅛ cup mayonnaise

1 egg

3 tablespoons butter, melted

1-2 lemon, cut into thin wedges for serving

Bearnaise sauce for serving, if desired

Directions:

To get started:

a)   Squeeze the crab meat to remove moisture;

b)   Preheat the oven to 425°F; and

c)   Butter a baking sheet.

Mix the mustard, seasoning, mayonnaise, and egg in a bowl. Refrigerate for 10 minutes.

Remove the mixture from the refrigerator, and add in the cracker crumbs. Continue mixing.

Pour the mixture over the crab and continue mixing.

Divide the mixture into 12, and then shape each dollop into a 1-inch thick circle.

Place the cakes on the baking sheet and drizzle some butter over each.

Bake for 15 to 20 minutes, until cakes are cooked through. Serve with lemon wedges and béarnaise sauce, if desired.

Nutrition: Calories: 200, Fat: 6 g, Carbs: 18 g, Protein: 18 g, Sodium: 502 mg

Olive Garden's Chicken and Shrimp Carbonara

Preparation Time: 35 minutes

Cooking Time: 40 minutes

Servings: 8

Ingredients:

Shrimp Marinade

¼ cup extra virgin olive oil

½ cup water

2 teaspoons Italian seasoning

1 tablespoon minced garlic

Chicken:

4 boneless and skinless chicken breasts cubed

1 egg mixed with 1 tablespoon cold water

½ cup panko bread crumbs

½ cup all-purpose flour

½ teaspoon salt

½ teaspoon black pepper

2 tablespoons olive oil

Carbonara sauce:

½ cup butter (1 stick)

3 tablespoons all-purpose flour

½ cup parmesan cheese, grated

2 cups heavy cream

2 cups milk

8 Canadian bacon slices, diced finely

¾ cup roasted red peppers, diced

Pasta:

1 teaspoon salt

14 ounces spaghetti or bucatini pasta (1 package)

Water to cook the pasta

Shrimp:

½ pound fresh medium shrimp, deveined and peeled

1-2 tablespoons olive oil for cooking

Directions:

Mix all the marinade ingredients together in a re-sealable container or bag and add the add shrimp. Refrigerate for at least 30 minutes.

To make the chicken: Mix the flour, salt, pepper, and panko bread crumbs into a shallow dish. Whisk the egg with 1 tablespoon of cold water in a second shallow dish. Dip the chicken into the breadcrumb mix and after in the egg wash, and again in the breadcrumb mix. Place on a plate and let rest until all the chicken is prepared.

Warm the olive oil over medium heat in a deep large skillet. Working in batches, add the chicken. Cook for 4 to 6 minutes per side or until the chicken is cooked through. Place the cooked chicken tenders on a plate lined with paper towels to absorb excess oil.

To make the pasta: Add water to large pot and bring to a boil. Add salt and cook the pasta according to package instructions about 10-15 minutes before the sauce is ready.

To make the shrimp: While the pasta is cooking, add olive oil to a skillet. Remove the shrimp from the marinate and shake off the excess marinade. Cook the shrimp until they turn pink, about 2-3 minutes.

To make the Carbonara sauce: in a large deep skillet, sauté the Canadian bacon with a bit of butter for 3-4 minutes over medium heat or until the bacon starts to caramelize. Add the garlic and sauté for 1 more minute. Remove bacon and garlic and set aside.

In the same skillet, let the butter melt and mix-in the flour. Gradually add the cream and milk and whisk until the sauce thickens. Add the cheese.

Reduce the heat to a simmer and keep the mixture simmering while you prepare the rest of the ingredients.

When you are ready to serve, add the drained pasta, bacon bits, roasted red peppers to sauce. Stir to coat. Add pasta evenly to each serving plate. Top with some chicken and shrimp. Garnish with fresh parsley Serve with fresh shredded Romano or Parmesan cheese

Nutrition: Calories: 1570, Fat: 113 g, Carbs: 84 g, Protein: 55 g, Sodium: 2400 mg

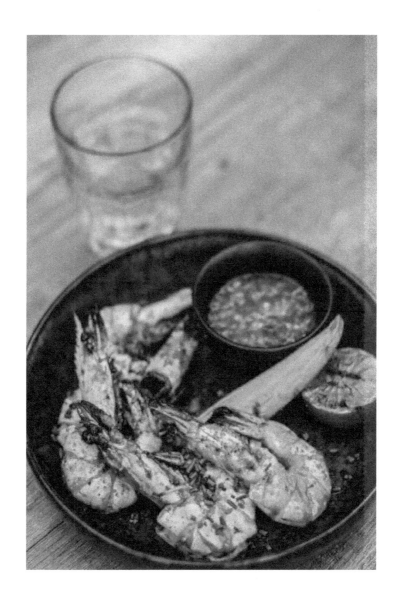

Bubba Gump Shrimp Company's Cajun Shrimp

Preparation Time: 5 minutes

Cooking Time: 15 minutes

Servings: 4

Ingredients:

2 teaspoons paprika

1 teaspoon dried thyme

½ teaspoon salt

¼ teaspoon nutmeg, ground

¼ teaspoon garlic powder

⅛ teaspoon cayenne pepper

1 tablespoon olive oil

1 pound fresh medium-sized shrimp, peeled, deveined

Directions:

Sauté all the ingredients (except for the shrimp) in oil for 30 seconds.

When the ingredients have heated up, add the shrimp and continue sautéing for 2 to 3 minutes.

When the shrimp is cooked entirely, transfer to a plate and serve.

Nutrition: Calories: 270, Fat: 234 g, Carbs: 169 g, Protein: 70 g, Sodium: 2878 mg

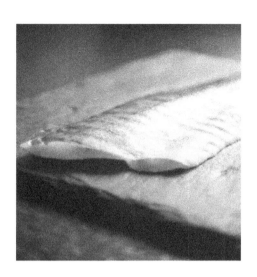

Herb Grilled Salmon

Preparation Time: 10 minutes

Cooking Time: 10 minutes

Servings: 4

Ingredients:

4 salmon steaks

Olive oil for brushing

Salt and pepper to taste

Lemon herb butter:

1 pound butter

1½ lemons (zest and juice but no seeds)

1 tablespoon fresh chopped herbs like basil and thyme

2 teaspoons fresh parsley, chopped

Directions:

To make the lemon herb butter, combine the butter, lemon zest, lemon juice and herbs in a food processor. Blend until smooth. Transfer to plastic wrap. Shape into a log and twist to seal. Chill in the refrigerator for up to three weeks.

Preheat a gas grill on medium heat or start a medium fire in a charcoal grill.

Brush the olive oil onto the fish fillets. Sprinkle with salt and pepper. Grill until fully cooked (when the salmon begins to change colors and becomes flaky).

Remove from the grill and top with the lemon herb butter. Serve.

Nutrition: Calories: 122, Fat: 23 g, Carbs: 33 g, Protein: 24 g, Sodium: 428 mg

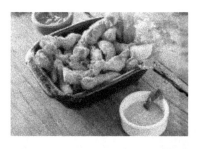
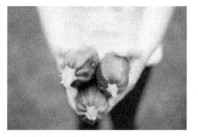
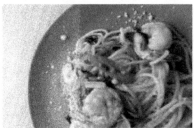

Fettuccine with Shrimp and Zucchini

Preparation Time: 10 minutes

Cooking Time: 7 minutes

Servings: 4

Ingredients:

1 pound dry fettuccine

½ cup extra-virgin olive oil

1 tablespoon garlic, chopped

2 tablespoons parsley, chopped

1 medium zucchini

1 pound large shrimp

1 cup dry white wine

¾ teaspoon salt

¾ teaspoon black pepper

¼ cup butter

6 lemon wedges

1 sprig parsley, chopped

Directions:

Slice zucchini into approximately 2×¼-inch sticks. Peel and devein shrimp.

Cook pasta according to package directions. Drain and set aside.

In a sauté pan, heat the oil over medium heat. Cook garlic and parsley for 1 minute.

Add the zucchini slices and cook for 1 minute. Add the shrimp, wine, salt, pepper, and butter. Stir and cook the shrimp for 5 minutes.

Toss the pasta into the saucepan. Mix well. Squeeze some lemon over the pasta. Serve.

Nutrition: Calories: 153, Fat: 24.5 g, Carbs: 16. 5 g

Protein: 35 g, Sodium: 645 mg

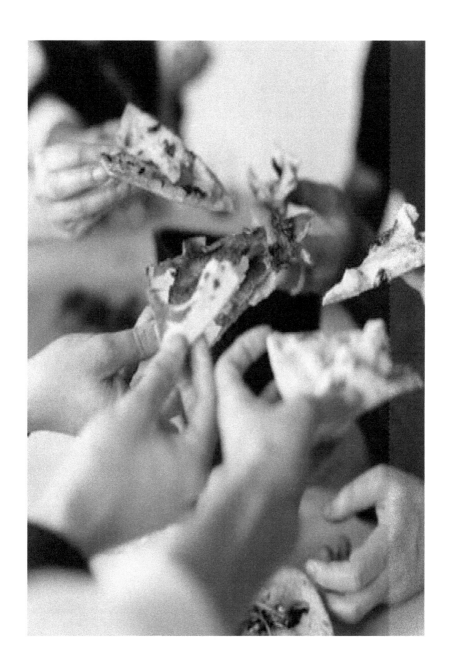

Dinner

Make-At-Home KFC Original Fried Chicken

Preparation Time: 20 minutes

Cooking Time: 40 minutes

Servings: 4

Ingredients:

Spice mix:

1 tablespoon paprika

2 teaspoons onion salt

1 teaspoon chili powder

1 teaspoon black pepper, ground

½ teaspoon celery salt

½ teaspoon dried sage

½ teaspoon garlic powder

½ teaspoon allspice, ground

½ teaspoon dried oregano

½ teaspoon dried basil

½ teaspoon dried marjoram

Chicken preparation:

1 whole chicken, cut into parts

2 quarts frying oil

1 egg white

1 ½ cups all-purpose flour

1 tablespoon brown sugar

1 tablespoon kosher salt

Directions:

Preheat oil in deep-fryer to 350°F.

In a bowl, mix together ingredients for the spice mix. Then, add flour, sugar, and salt. Mix well until fully blended.

Coat each chicken piece with egg white, then the flour breading. Make sure that the chicken pieces are well-coated.

Transfer to a plate and allow chicken to dry for about 5 minutes.

Deep-fry breasts and wings together for about 12 minutes or until the temperature on a meat thermometer inserted in the breast's thickest part reads 165 °F. Do the same with legs and thighs. Usually these parts take 1-2 minutes more to cook.

Transfer pieces onto a plate lined with paper towels.

Serve.

Nutrition: Calories 418 Total, Fat 22 g, Carbs 41 g, Protein 15 g, Sodium 1495 mg

Copycat California Pizza Kitchen's California Club Pizza

Preparation Time: 5 minutes

Cooking Time: 12 minutes

Servings: 4

Ingredients:

1 ball pizza dough

2 tablespoons olive oil

1 chicken breast, cooked and chopped into bite-sized pieces

4 slices of bacon, cooked and cut into bite-sized pieces

1 cup mozzarella cheese, grated

1½ cups arugula

2 tablespoons mayonnaise

1 tomato, sliced

1 avocado, peeled and cut into 8 slices

Directions:

Preheat pizza stone in oven to 425°F.

Using a rolling pin, flatten pizza dough until it is about 12 to 14 inches in diameter. Brush olive oil in a thin and even layer on top. Add chicken, bacon, and mozzarella in layers evenly across pizza dough.

Place onto pizza stone and bake for about 10 to 12 minutes or until cheese melts and crust is slightly brown. Remove from oven and set aside.

In a bowl, add arugula and mayonnaise. Mix well. Top cooked pizza with tomato, arugula mixture, and avocado.

Serve warm.

Nutrition: Calories 456, Total fat 32 g, Saturated fat 8 g, Carbs 18 g, Sugar 2 g, Fibers 4 g, Protein 26 g, Sodium 625 mg

Oriental Salad from Applebee's

Preparation Time: 15 minutes

Cooking Time: 5 minutes

Servings: 6

Ingredients:

3 tablespoons honey

1½ tablespoons rice wine vinegar

¼ cup mayonnaise

1 teaspoon Dijon mustard

⅛ teaspoon sesame oil

3 cups vegetable oil, for frying

2 chicken breasts, cut into thin strips

1 egg

1 cup milk

1 cup flour

1 cup breadcrumbs

1 teaspoon salt

¼ teaspoon pepper

3 cups romaine lettuce, diced

½ cup red cabbage, diced

½ cup napa cabbage, diced

1 carrot, grated

¼ cup cucumber, diced

3 tablespoons sliced almonds

¼ cup dry chow mein

Directions:

To make the dressing, add honey, rice wine vinegar, mayonnaise, Dijon mustard, and sesame oil to a blender. Mix until well combined. Store in refrigerator until ready to serve.

Heat oil in a deep pan over medium-high heat.

As oil warms, whisk together egg and milk in a bowl. In another bowl, add flour, breadcrumbs, salt, and pepper. Mix well.

Dredge chicken strips in egg mixture, then in the flour mixture. Make sure the chicken is coated evenly on all sides. Shake off any excess.

Deep fry chicken strips for about 3 to 4 minutes until thoroughly cooked and lightly brown. Transfer onto a plate lined with paper towels to drain and cool. Work in batches, if necessary.

Chop strips into small, bite-size pieces once cool enough to handle.

Next, prepare salad by adding romaine, red cabbage, napa cabbage, carrots, and cucumber to a serving bowl. Top with chicken pieces, almonds, and chow mein. Drizzle prepared dressing on top.

Serve immediately.

Nutrition: Calories 384, Total fat 13 g, Saturated fat 3 g, Carbs 40 g, Sugar 13 g, Fibers 2 g, Protein 27 g, Sodium 568 mg

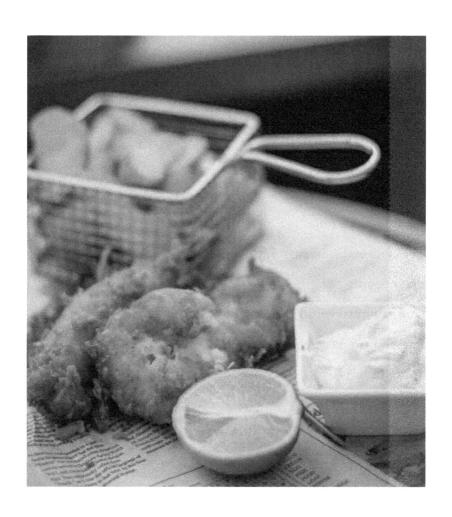

Other Restaurant Favorites I

Chick-fil-A Chicken Nuggets with Honey Mustard Dipping Sauce

Preparation Time: 15 minutes

Cooking Time: 15 minutes

Servings: 4

Ingredients:

1 egg

¾ cup milk

¼ cup dill pickle juice

2 large chicken breasts, cut into bite-sized pieces

Salt and pepper to taste

1¼ cups all-purpose flour

2 tablespoons powdered sugar

2 teaspoons salt

1 teaspoon pepper

½ cup canola oil

½ cup plain Greek yogurt

1½ tablespoons yellow mustard

1 tablespoon Dijon mustard

2 tablespoons honey

Directions:

Mix egg, milk, and pickle juice in a bowl until well combined. Season chicken pieces with salt and pepper and then add to egg mixture. Refrigerate for at least 2 hours to marinate.

In another bowl, add flour, powdered sugar, salt, and pepper. Mix well until combined. Transfer chicken from marinade into flour mixture. Toss and fold to coat thoroughly and evenly on all sides.

Heat ½ cup oil in a large pan over medium-high heat. The oil is hot enough if it sizzles when you sprinkle a little of the flour mixture on top but if it pops, it's too hot. Lower temperature if this happens.

One at a time, slowly add chicken into hot oil. Allow spacing between pieces. Deep fry pieces for about 3 to 4 minutes until one side is lightly brown. Using tongs, turn pieces over and continue cooking for another 3 to 4 minutes. Transfer to a plate lined with paper towels.

To make the dipping sauce, combine Greek yogurt, both mustards, and honey in a bowl. Mix well. Serve on the side with hot chicken pieces.

Nutrition: Calories 395, Total fat 6 g, Saturated fat 2 g, Carbs 45 g, Sugar 16 g, Fibers 2 g, Protein 39 g, Sodium 1434 mg

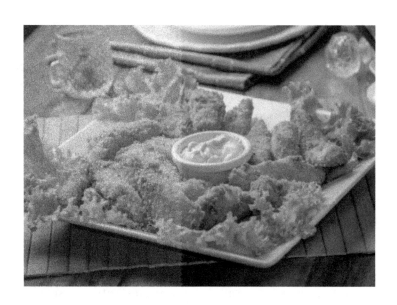

Red Lobster's Garlic Shrimp Scampi

Preparation Time: 15 minutes

Cooking Time: 15 minutes

Servings: 4

Ingredients:

1 pound shrimp, peeled and deveined

Salt and pepper to taste

1 tablespoon olive oil

3 garlic cloves, finely chopped

1½ white wine

2 tablespoons lemon juice

¼ teaspoon dried basil

¼ teaspoon dried oregano

¼ teaspoon dried rosemary

¼ teaspoon dried thyme

½ cup butter

2 tablespoons parsley leaves, minced

¼ cup Parmesan cheese, shredded (optional)

Directions:

Flavor shrimp with salt and pepper.

In a pan with heated oil, sauté shrimp on medium-high heat for about 2 minutes or until color changes to pink. Transfer onto a plate for later.

In the same pan, sauté garlic for 30 seconds or until aromatic. Pour in white wine and lemon juice. Stir, then bring to a boil. Adjust heat to medium-low and cook for an additional 4 minutes. Mix in basil, oregano, rosemary, and thyme. Then, add butter gradually. Mix until completely melted and blended with other ingredients. Remove from heat.

Return shrimp to pan and add parsley. Taste and adjust seasoning with salt and pepper as needed.

Sprinkle Parmesan on top, if desired. Serve.

Nutrition: Calories 448, Total Fat 29 g, Carbs 3 g, Protein 26 g, Sodium 362 mg

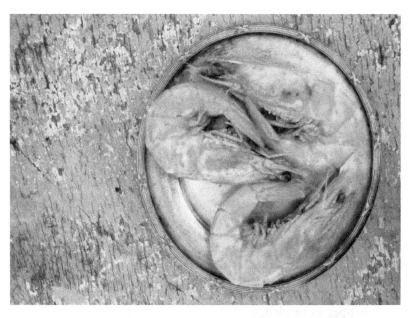

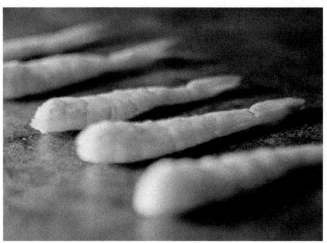

Bonefish Grill's Bang Bang Shrimp

Preparation Time: 5 minutes

Cooking Time: 5 minutes

Servings: 4

Ingredients:

½ cup mayonnaise

¼ cup Thai sweet chili sauce

3-5 drops hot chili sauce (or more if you like it spicier)

½ cup cornstarch

1 pound small shrimp, peeled and deveined

1½ cups vegetable oil

Directions:

To make the sauce, combine mayonnaise with Thai chili sauce and hot chili sauce in a bowl.

In a separate bowl, add cornstarch. Toss shrimp in cornstarch until well-coated.

Heat oil in a wok. Working in batches, fry shrimp until golden brown, about 2-3 minutes. Transfer onto a plate lined with paper towels to drain excess oil.

Serve shrimp in a bowl with sauce drizzled on top.

Nutrition: Calories 274, Total Fat 11 g, Carbs 26 g, Protein 16 g, Sodium 1086 mg

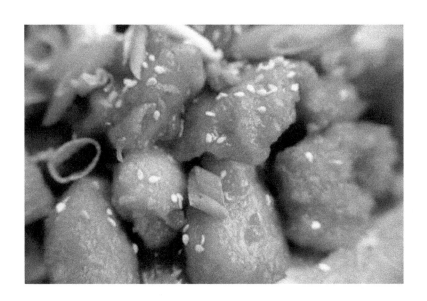

Chi-Chi's Seafood Chimichanga

Preparation Time: 10 minutes

Cooking Time: 30 minutes

Servings: 6

Ingredients:

4 tablespoons butter

4 tablespoons flour

½ teaspoon butter

2 dashes black pepper, ground

2 cups milk

8 ounces jack cheese, shredded

1 16-ounce package crab meat, flaked

1 cup cottage cheese

¼ cup Parmesan cheese

1 egg

1 tablespoon dried parsley flakes

¼ teaspoon onion powder

1 tablespoon lemon juice

Shredded lettuce for serving

¼ cup sliced green onions for garnish

Directions:

Preheat oven to 375°F.

To make the sauce, heat butter in a pan on medium heat. Add flour, salt, and pepper. Mix, then pour in milk. Stirring often, cook until sauce is thick then simmer for an additional 1 minute.

Turn off heat and stir in jack cheese until completely blended into sauce.

In a bowl, combine crab meat, cottage and Parmesan cheese, egg, parsley, and onion powder. Heat tortillas in microwave for 10 seconds or until warm. Wet bottom side of tortilla and add crab meat mixture on top. Fold tortilla to wrap filling.

Coat baking sheet with cooking spray. Bake chimichangas for about 25 minutes.

Reheat sauce until warm. Mix in lemon juice and stir until blended.

Transfer chimichangas to plates over a bed of shredded lettuce, if desired. Top with sauce and garnish with green onions before serving.

Nutrition: Calories 794, Total Fat 33 g, Carbs 77 g, Protein 44 g, Sodium 1932 mg

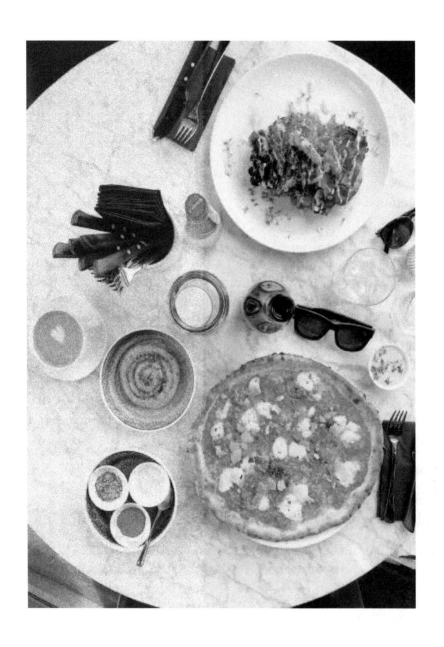

Red Lobster's Copycat Lobster Pizza

Preparation Time: 15 minutes

Cooking Time: 5 minutes

Servings: 1

Ingredients:

1 10-inch flour tortillas

1 ounce roasted garlic butter

2 tablespoons Parmesan cheese, shredded

1/2 cup fresh Roma tomatoes, finely chopped

2 tablespoons fresh basil, cut into thin strips

2 ounces lobster meat, chopped

½ cup Italian cheese blend, grated

Vegetable oil for coating

Dash salt and pepper

Fresh lemon juice for serving

Directions:

Preheat oven to 450°F.

Coat one side of tortilla with garlic butter. Top with Parmesan cheese, tomatoes, basil, lobster meat, and Italian cheese blend in that order. Set aside.

Prepare a pizza pan. Apply a light coat of vegetable oil and cover with a dash of salt and pepper. Transfer pizza onto pan. Bake for about 5 minutes.

Cut into slices and drizzle with lemon juice.

Serve.

Nutrition: Calories 339, Total Fat 10 g, Carbs 41 g, Protein 22 g, Sodium 890 mg

Bonefish Grill's Skewered Shrimp with Pan-Asian Glaze

Preparation Time: 5 minutes

Cooking Time: 10 minutes

Servings: 4

Ingredients:

¼ ketchup

¼ cup oyster sauce

1 tablespoon soy sauce

1 tablespoon water

¾ tablespoon lemon juice

1 tablespoon extra-virgin olive oil, plus more

1 tablespoon fresh ginger, peeled and finely chopped

1 tablespoon sugar

1 tablespoon honey

1 pound shrimp, peeled, deveined, and skewered

Preparation:

In a bowl, add ketchup, oyster sauce, soy sauce, water, and lemon juice. Mix well.

Add olive oil to a deep pan over medium heat. Once hot, stir fry ginger for about 1 minute until aromatic. Pour in ketchup mixture. Once simmering, lower heat to medium-low. Add sugar and honey. Cook for 1 minute, stirring frequently. Remove from heat. Set aside.

Preheat grill over high heat. Coat top with olive oil. Dry shrimp with a paper towel, then season all sides with salt and pepper. Add to grill and cook for 1 to 2 minutes until color changes. Turn shrimp, then coat cooked side with prepared glaze mixture. Grill until bottom side is cooked, then turn again. Apply glaze to other side. Remove from grill.

Serve.

Nutrition: Calories 199, Total fat 5 g, Saturated fat 1 g, Carbs 14 g, Sugar 8 g, Fibers 0 g, Protein 24 g, Sodium 750 mg

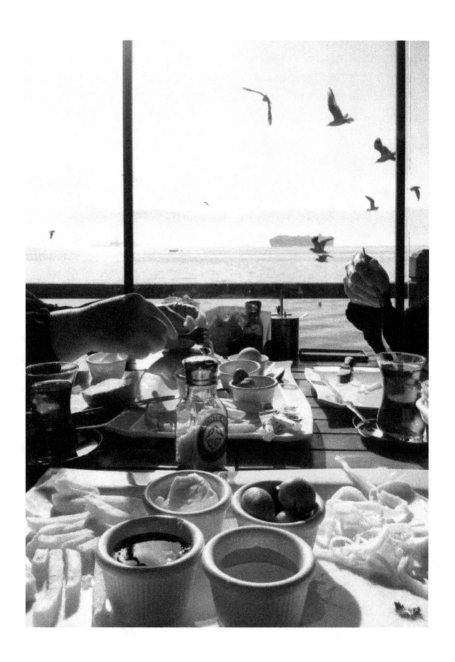

DIY Red Hook's Lobster Pound

Preparation Time: 10 minutes

Cooking Time: 10 minutes

Servings: 2

Ingredients:

2 large egg yolks

1 teaspoon Dijon mustard

4 teaspoons fresh lemon juice, plus more

1 cup vegetable oil

Coarse salt and ground pepper, to taste

¾ pounds lobster meat, cooked and chopped into 1-inch cubes

2 top-split hot dog rolls

2 tablespoons butter, melted

Iceberg lettuce, shredded

1 scallion, finely sliced

Paprika, to taste

Directions:

To make the DIY mayonnaise, add egg yolks, mustard, and lemon juice to a food processor. Process until fully mixed. Then, while still processing, gradually add oil until mixture thickens and becomes cloudy. Add salt and pepper.

Transfer to a bowl and cover. Set aside.

Prepare lobster filling by combining lobster pieces, prepared mayonnaise, lemon juice, salt, and pepper in a bowl.

Heat griddle. Apply butter to insides of hotdog rolls. Place rolls to grill butter side down, and cook until golden brown.

Assemble lobster rolls by layering lettuce, lobster and mayonnaise mixture, scallions, and paprika. Repeat for 2nd lobster roll.

Serve.

Nutrition: Calories 1746, Total fat 135 g, Saturated fat 90 g, Carbs 49 g, Sugar 9 g, Fibers 5 g, Protein 92 g, Sodium 2299 mg

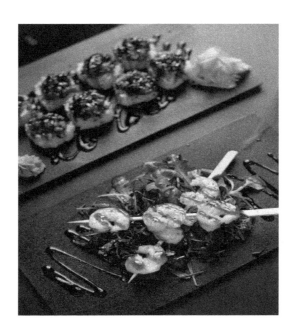

Copycat Bubba Gum's Coconut Shrimp

Preparation Time: 5 minutes

Cooking Time: 20 minutes

Servings: 2

Ingredients:

Oil, for deep frying

½ pound medium raw shrimp, peeled and deveined

¾ cup pancake mix

¾ cup wheat beer

¼ cup all-purpose flour

¼ teaspoon seasoning salt

¼ teaspoon cayenne pepper

337

¼ teaspoon garlic powder

1 cup shredded coconut

Sauce:

¼ cup orange marmalade

½ teaspoon Cajun seasoning

Directions:

Preheat deep fryer to 350°F.

Run cold water over shrimp then dry using a paper towel. Set aside.

Prepare 3 bowls for the different coatings. In the 1st bowl, combine pancake mix and beer. In the 2nd, combine flour, seasoning salt, cayenne pepper, and garlic powder. For the 3rd bowl, add coconut.

One at a time, dredge shrimp into 1st bowl, shaking excess flour, then into the 2nd bowl followed by the 3rd.

Deep fry shrimp for about 45 to 60 seconds until lightly brown. Then, transfer onto a plate lined with paper towels to drain.

Prepare dipping sauce by combining sauce ingredients in a bowl.

Serve shrimp with dipping sauce on the side.

Nutrition: Calories 609, Total fat 15 g, Saturated fat 12 g, Carbs 84 g, Sugar 35 g, Fibers 6 g, Protein 32 g, Sodium 1555 mg

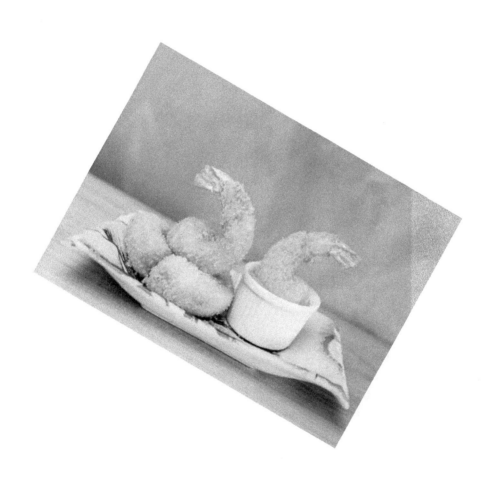

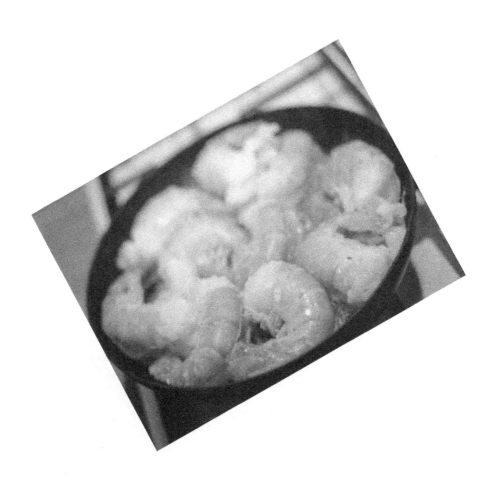

T.G.I. Friday's Black Bean Soup

Preparation Time: 10 minutes

Cooking Time: 1 hour 15 minutes

Servings: 6

Ingredients:

2 tablespoons vegetable oil

¾ cup white onion, diced

¾ cup celery, diced

½ cup carrot, diced

¼ cup green bell pepper, diced

2 tablespoons garlic, minced

4 15-ounce cans black beans, rinsed

4 cups chicken stock

2 tablespoons apple cider vinegar

2 teaspoons chili powder

½ teaspoon cayenne pepper

½ teaspoon cumin

½ teaspoon salt

¼ teaspoon hickory liquid smoke

Directions:

In a pan, sauté the onion, celery, carrot, bell pepper, and garlic in the heated oil for 15 minutes over low heat. Make sure to keep the vegetables from burning.

While the vegetables are cooking, strain and wash the black beans.

Add 3 cups of the washed beans and a cup of chicken stock to a food processor and purée until smooth.

When the onion mixture is cooked, add the rest of the ingredients (including the bean purée) to the pan.

Bring everything to a boil, then lower the heat and allow the mixture to simmer for another 50 to 60 minutes.

Transfer the soup to bowls and serve.

Nutrition: Calories 392.5, Total Fat 7.8 g, Carbs 59.3 g

Protein 23 g, Sodium 458.9 mg

Olive Garden's Minestrone Soup

Preparation Time: 5 minutes

Cooking Time: 40 minutes

Servings: 8

Ingredients:

3 tablespoons olive oil

½ cup green beans, sliced

¼ cup celery, diced

1 cup white onion diced)

1 zucchini, diced

4 teaspoons minced garlic

4 cups vegetable broth

1 can (15 ounces each) red kidney beans, drained

2 cans (15 ounces each) small white beans, drained

1 can (14 ounce) tomatoes, diced

1 carrot, peeled and diced

2 tablespoons fresh Italian parsley, chopped finely

1½ teaspoons dried oregano

1½ teaspoons salt

½ teaspoon ground black pepper

½ teaspoon dried basil

¼ teaspoon dried thyme

3 cups hot water

4 cups fresh baby spinach

½ cup small shell pasta

Shredded parmesan cheese for serving

Directions:

Chop and mince the ingredients as specified.

Sauté the green beans, celery, onion, zucchini, and garlic in olive oil in a soup pot until the onions become translucent.

Add in the rest of the ingredients, except the beans, pasta, and spinach leaves, and bring the mixture to a boil.

When the mixture is boiling, add in the beans, spinach and pasta. Reduce the heat and allow to simmer for another 20 minutes.

Ladle into a bowl, sprinkle with parmesan if desired, and serve.

Nutrition: Calories 353.5, Total Fat 6.3 g, Carbs 57.8 g, Protein 19.2 g, Sodium 471.7 mg

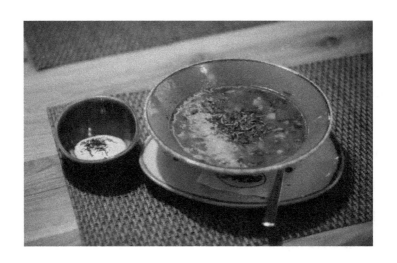

Panera Bread's Vegetarian Summer Corn Chowder

Preparation Time: 10 minutes

Cooking Time: 45 minutes

Servings: 6

Ingredients:

2 tablespoons olive oil

1 tablespoon unsalted butter

1 medium red onion, diced

3 tablespoons all-purpose flour

2 russet potatoes, diced

5 cups unsalted vegetable stock

½ cup red bell pepper, diced

½ cup green bell pepper, diced

4 cups whole corn kernels

¼ teaspoon black pepper, ground

1 cup half-and-half cream

Salt and pepper to taste

Chives, thinly sliced, for garnish

Bacon bits, for garnish

Directions:

Sauté the onion in butter and oil over low heat. When the onion becomes translucent, add in the flour and cook for another 5 minutes.

Dice the potatoes into quarter-inch cubes and add it to the simmering mixture. Add the broth, then turn the heat up and bring the mixture to a boil.

Reduce the heat to medium and continue simmering for 15 minutes.

Dice the bell peppers into quarter-inch cubes and add them to the mixture. Also add in the corn, pepper, cream, salt, and pepper, and allow the mixture to simmer for another 15 minutes.

Transfer the soup into a bowl and garnish with chives and bacon, if desired.

Nutrition: Calories 320, Total Fat 20 g, Carbs 34 g, Protein 5 g, Sodium 1310 mg

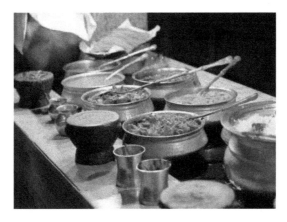

Hostess® Twinkies

Preparation Time: 15 minutes

Cooking Time: 55 minutes

Servings: 2

Ingredients:

For Cake:

7 egg whites

½ teaspoon tartar cream

2 cups flour

1 ½ cups sugar

1 tablespoon baking powder

7 egg yolks

½ cup vegetable oil

¾ cup cold water

2 teaspoons vanilla

½ teaspoon salt

For Filling:

6 tablespoons flour (rounded)

1 ½ cups Butter Flavor Crisco

1 ½ cups sugar

1 cup cold milk (scant)

2 teaspoons vanilla

Directions:

Preheat your oven to 350 F.

Mix flour with baking powder, sugar & salt in a large sized bowl; mix well. Make a well in the middle & add in the oil, vanilla, cold water & egg yolks. Using a large spoon, beat well until smooth; set aside.

Beat whites with cream of tartar until stiff peaks appear. Transfer on top of the egg yolk batter & fold in until combined.

Transfer to a 10x14" pan, ungreased & bake for 45 to 50 minutes. Let cool for couple of minutes and then turn upside down into another pan. Let cool, then run a knife around the edges. Remove & cut in half.

Now, for the filling, mix flour together with Butter Flavor Crisco & sugar; beat for 4 to 5 minutes on high & then gradually add in vanilla & milk. Beat on high again for 3 to 5 more minutes. Spread the mixture between 2 even layers & cut it into 3x1" size & wrap them individually

Nutrition: Calories: 3391 kcal, Protein: 41.21 g, Fat: 239.44 g, Carbohydrates: 273.27 g

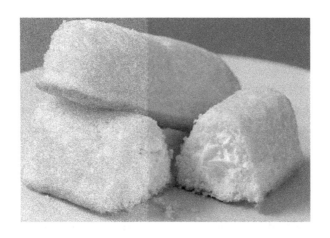

Hostess® Sno Balls®

Preparation Time: 15 minutes

Cooking Time: 1 hour & 10 minutes

Servings: 10

Ingredients:

For the Cake:

3 eggs

1 stick butter, unsalted, softened

2 teaspoons baking soda

1 teaspoon of vanilla extract

2 cups all-purpose flour

1/3 cup cocoa powder

2 cups sugar

1 ½ cups milk

½ teaspoon salt

For the Frosting:

3 drops of red food coloring

1 ½ cups sugar

6 egg whites

1 teaspoon cream of tarter

2 cups coconut, shredded

1 teaspoon coconut extract

2 teaspoons vanilla extract

1/3 cup water

Directions:

For the Cake:

Cream butter with the sugar & then gradually add in vanilla & eggs. Whisk flour together with the cocoa, baking soda & salt in a separate large sized bowl.

Add half of the dry mixture to sugar/butter mixture & then add in the milk and the remaining dry mixture.

Scoop everything into a lightly greased muffin tin & bake for 15 minutes at 350 F. Allow it to cool for some time at room temperature.

Cut a cone from the bottom of every cake & trim the tip off.

For the Filling:

Beat the egg whites well until soft peaks form, for couple of minutes.

Combine sugar together with cream of tartar & water in a small sized saucepan; bring everything to a boil, over moderate heat settings. Remove the pan from heat & let cool a bit at room temperature.

Gradually pour the syrup into the egg whites and then add in vanilla & coconut extract.

Whip until the mixture is thickened, for 10 more minutes. Process the coconut in a food processor. If desired, feel free to add food coloring during this process.

Replace the cap of the cake; leaving it upside down for the frosting.

Generously coat the bottom & sides with a layer of frosting and then add in the coconut sprinkles.

Nutrition: Calories: 400 kcal, Protein: 9.56 g, Carbohydrates: 59.84 g

Other Restaurant Favorites II

Hostess® Cupcakes

Preparation Time: 15 minutes

Cooking Time: 1 hour 15 minutes

Servings: 10

Ingredients:

For Cupcakes:

1 ½ cups sugar

2 cups flour

¾ cup Dutch process cocoa

1 teaspoon of baking powder

1 ½ teaspoons of baking soda

½ teaspoon salt

2 eggs

1 cup oil

¾ cup buttermilk

1 teaspoon vanilla

¾ cup hot coffee

For Ganache:

¾ cup cream

7 ounces chocolate

For Filling:

4 tablespoons butter

1 cup powdered sugar

2 teaspoons vanilla

1 cup marshmallow crème

For Icing:

½ stick butter

1 cup powdered sugar

½ teaspoon vanilla

½ -1 tablespoon milk

Directions:

Preheat your oven to 350 F. Sift flour together with Dutch process cocoa, sugar, baking soda, baking powder & salt in a large sized bowl. Beat eggs together with oil, vanilla & buttermilk in a separate bowl, and then add the mixture into the dry ingredients. Beat in the warm coffee.

Pour the mixture into the lined muffin cups & fill them approximately 2/3 full; bake for 18 to 20 minutes at 350 F. Remove from oven & let cool a bit at room temperature. Beat all the filling ingredients together in a medium sized bowl. Fill a large sized piping bag. When you can easily handle the cupcakes, press their tip into the middle & squeeze one or two tablespoons of cream filling into the middle. Repeat the process for all the cupcakes.

Over medium heat settings in a large saucepan; heat the cream until the cream is hot & just begins to boil, stirring frequently. Transfer the cream immediately on top of the chocolate; whisk until smooth. Spread the slightly cooled but warm ganache on top of the filled cupcakes.

Whip all the icing ingredients together until smooth; if required, feel free to add more of milk. Fill a piping bag & pipe on the curls.

Nutrition: Calories: 609 kcal, Protein: 7.19 g, Fat: 33.47 g, Carbohydrates: 73.72 g

Starbucks® Iced Lemon Pound Cake

Preparation Time: 15 minutes

Cooking Time: 1 hour

Servings: 12

Ingredients:

For Cake:

6 tablespoons lemon juice, freshly squeezed

1 package lemon pudding mix, non-instant (4.3 ounce)

8 ounces sour cream

1 package yellow cake mix (18.25 ounce)

½ cup milk

4 eggs, large

½ cup vegetable oil

For Icing:

3 tablespoons lemon juice, freshly squeezed or more to taste

2 ½ cups confectioners' sugar

Directions:

Lightly grease two loaf pans & preheat your oven to 350 F in advance.

Now, mix cake mix together with eggs, oil, pudding mix, sour cream, 6 tablespoons of the lemon juice, and milk in a stand mixer; beat for couple of minutes & then transfer the mixture into already prepared greased loaf pans.

Bake for 45 to 50 minutes, until a toothpick should come out clean. Before removing the cake from pans, let cool in the pans for couple of minutes & then transfer on a wire rack to completely cool.

Now, whisk the icing ingredients together in a medium sized bowl until smooth, for couple of minutes; evenly spoon the mixture over the loaves & let set for half an hour, before you slice them into pieces.

Nutrition: Calories: 414 kcal, Protein: 3.98 g, Fat: 15.39 g, Carbohydrates: 66.83 g

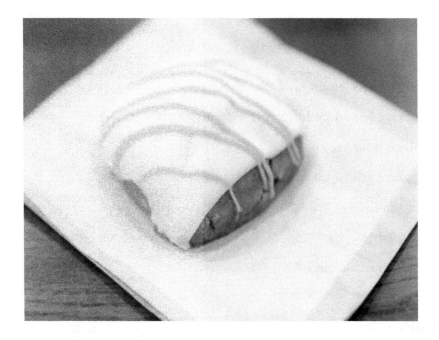

Starbucks® Banana Bread

Preparation Time: 15 minutes

Cooking Time: 50 minutes

Servings: 8

Ingredients:

3 ripe bananas, medium-large, mashed

1/3 cup chopped walnuts (in addition to 1/2 cup)

1 egg, large

2 cups flour

½ cup plus 1/3 cup walnuts, chopped

1 teaspoon baking soda

½ teaspoon vanilla extract

2 tablespoons buttermilk

½ cup vegetable oil

1 1/8 cups sugar

¼ teaspoon salt

Directions:

Lightly grease a 9x5x3" loaf pan with the oil, dust with the flour & then preheat your oven to 325 F.

Blend baking soda together with flour & salt; set aside. Now, mix egg with vegetable oil & sugar until combined well.

Gradually add flour mixture to the egg mixture; blend well & then, add in the mashed bananas, vanilla & buttermilk; mix well. Fold approximately ½ cup of the chopped walnuts & transfer the batter into already prepared loaf pan.

Top the batter with the leftover walnuts. Bake until a toothpick comes out clean, for 50 to 60 minutes.

Nutrition: Calories: 350 kcal, Protein: 4.96 g, Fat: 19.94 g, Carbohydrates: 39.37 g

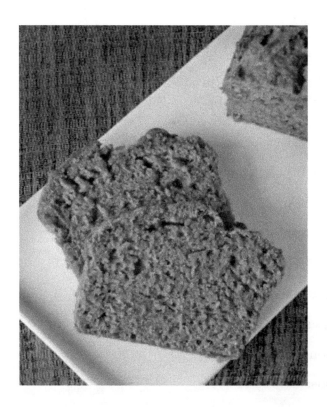

Starbucks® Vanilla Bean Scone

Preparation Time: 25 minutes

Cooking Time: 15 minutes

Servings: 16

Ingredients:

For Scones:

½ cup sugar

2 teaspoon vanilla extract

½ cup butter, cold, cubed

2 ½ cup all-purpose flour

½ cup heavy cream

1 tablespoon baking powder

½ vanilla bean, scraped

1 egg, large

¼ teaspoon salt

For Glaze:

6-7 tablespoon Heavy Cream

½ Vanilla Bean, scraped

1 teaspoon Vanilla Extract

3 cups powdered sugar

Directions:

Line a large baking sheet either with a silicone mat or parchment paper & preheat your oven to 400 F in advance.

Combine flour together with baking powder, salt & sugar. Pulse in a food processor or whisk until evenly mixed.

Add butter & pulse in a food processor or cut in using a pastry cutter until the mixture looks like a cornmeal texture.

Whisk cream together with egg, vanilla extract & scraping in a separate bowl.

Add liquid to the flour mixture & stir well using your hands until the dough forms a ball or pulse in a food processor until just combined.

Place the dough onto a lightly floured surface & then briefly knead until the dough comes together; roll the dough out to approximately ½ inch thickness.

Make 8 squares or rectangles from the dough & then cut each one diagonally & then create 32 small scones on the other.

Place them onto already prepared large sized baking sheet & bake or until the edges start to get golden brown, for 10 to 12 minutes.

Transfer the cooked scones to a cooling rack & let completely cool.

In the meantime; whisk the glaze ingredients together in a large sized bowl, keep adding one tablespoon of the cream until you get your desired thickness. Dip the cooled scones in the glaze & then place them onto cooling rack again until harden.

Nutrition: Calories: 247 kcal, Protein: 2.45 g, Fat: 9.87 g, Carbohydrates: 37.16 g

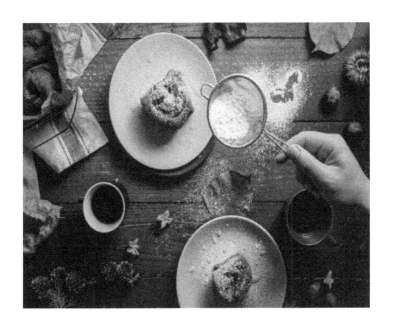

Starbucks® Pumpkin Scone

Preparation Time: 20 minutes

Cooking Time: 30 minutes

Servings: 6

Ingredients:

For Scones:

2 cups all-purpose flour

½ teaspoon each ground cinnamon & ground nutmeg

3 tablespoons half & half

1 tablespoon baking powder

¼ teaspoon each ground cloves & ground ginger

1 egg, large

6 tablespoons butter, cold

½ cup pumpkin, canned

7 tablespoons sugar

½ teaspoon salt

For Powdered Sugar Glaze:

2 tablespoons whole milk

1 cup plus 1 tablespoon powdered sugar

For Spiced Glaze

1 cup powdered sugar

3 tablespoons powdered sugar

2 tablespoons whole milk

¼ teaspoon ground cinnamon

1/8 teaspoon ground nutmeg

1 pinch of each ginger & ground cloves

Directions:

To Prepare the Scones:

Lightly oil a large sized baking sheet lined with a parchment paper & preheat your oven to 425 F.

Now, in a large sized bowl; combine flour together with baking powder, spices, salt & sugar; mix well. Cut the butter into the dry ingredients using a fork, pastry knife, or a food processor, until no obvious chunks of the butter & the mixture is crumbly; set aside.

Whisk pumpkin together with egg & half and half in a separate medium sized bowl. Mix wet ingredients with the dry ingredients; fold well & shape the dough into a ball.

Pat the dough out onto a lightly floured surface & make a 1" thick rectangle (approximately 3 inches wide & 9 inches long). Make three equal portions from the dough by slicing it twice through the width, using a pizza cutter or a large knife. Cut the slices diagonally until you get 6 triangular slices of the dough. Place them onto already prepared baking sheet & bake until turn lightly brown, for 12 to 15 minutes. Place them on a wire rack and let completely cool.

For the Plain Glaze:

Mix 2 tablespoon of milk together with the powdered sugar; mix well until completely smooth.

When you can handle the scones easily, paint the plain glaze on top of each scone using a brush.

For the Spiced Icing:

Combine the entire spicing ingredient together & drizzle this thicker icing on top of each scone; leave the icing for an hour and let dry, before serving. Drizzle with a whisk using a squirt bottle.

Nutrition: Calories: 507 kcal, Protein: 8.02 g, Fat: 17.69 g, Carbohydrates: 80.83 g

Starbucks® Coffee Cake

Preparation Time: 15 minutes

Cooking Time: 1 hour & 15 minutes

Servings: 8

Ingredients:

For the Batter

2 cups all-purpose flour

½ cup granulated sugar

2 eggs, large

1 cup softened butter

¾ cup packed sugar, light brown

1 ½ teaspoons vanilla

1/3 cup half & half

1 teaspoon of baking powder

¼ teaspoon salt

For Topping:

1 cup packed sugar, light brown

½ cup chopped pecans

1 cup all-purpose flour

½ cup softened butter

1 teaspoon cinnamon

Directions:

Preheat your oven to 325 F.

In a medium sized bowl; combine a cup of the flour with a stick of softened butter, brown sugar & 1 teaspoon of the cinnamon; mix well the mixture looks like moist sand. Add in half cup of pecans.

Now, using an electric mixer; cream 1 cup of butter together with ½ cup of granulated sugar & ¾ cup of light brown sugar until smooth & fluffy, in a large sized bowl. Add vanilla & eggs; mix well.

Combine flour together with baking powder & salt in a separate bowl. Combine the dry mixture with moist ingredients a small quantity at a time & then add in half & half; mix well.

Spoon the batter into a baking pan (9x13") lightly buttered & dusted with coating of flour.

Sprinkle the crumb topping on top of the batter. Ensure that the topping covers the batter completely.

Bake until the edges start to turn light brown, for 50 minutes. Let cool at room temperature & then slice into pieces.

Nutrition: Calories: 650 kcal, Protein: 6.71 g, Fat: 40.7 g, Carbohydrates: 66.09 g

Starbucks® Pumpkin Spice Latte

Preparation Time: 15 minutes

Cooking Time: 10 minutes

Servings: 1

Ingredients:

1 teaspoon vanilla simple syrup

1 cup coffee or 2 espresso shots

1 tablespoon pumpkin spice syrup

1 cup milk

For Garnish:

Whipped cream

Equal parts of pumpkin spice (ginger, cinnamon, ground clove, and nutmeg)

Directions:

Add milk together with vanilla syrup & pumpkin spice syrup into a microwave safe jar attached with a lid or a mason jar. Seal & shake until the milk is double in volume & frothy. Remove the lid & microwave until the milk is steamed, for a minute or two.

Transfer the hot milk either into coffee or espresso & top it first with the whipped cream & then a pinch of pumpkin spice.

Nutrition: Calories: 210 kcal, Protein: 8.3 g, Fat: 9.13 g, Carbohydrates: 25 g

Starbucks® Cranberry Bliss Bars

Preparation Time: 10 minutes

Cooking Time: 2 hours & 35 minutes

Servings: 40

Ingredients:

For Bars:

¾ cup white chocolate chips

2 sticks very soft butter (1 cup)

¾ cup dried cranberries (craisins)

3 eggs, large

2/3 cup to 1 cup brown sugar

2 cups all-purpose flour

1/3 cup granulated sugar

2 teaspoons vanilla or orange extract

1 ½ teaspoons baking powder

1 teaspoon ground ginger

For Topping:

½ teaspoon canola oil

1/3 cup white chocolate chips

1 -2 tablespoon orange rind, grated

1/3 cup chopped Craisins

For Frosting:

3 cups confectioners' sugar

1 teaspoon vanilla or orange extract

3 ounces softened cream cheese

2 tablespoons softened butter

Directions:

Line in a 10x15" pan with the parchment paper & preheat your oven to 350 F.

Beat softened butter together with sugars using an electric mixer, until light, for 3 to 5 minutes; gently blend in the orange extract and eggs (don't overbeat the eggs). Add in the flour, ginger & baking powder; beat for a short time. Add in the chips & cranberries, keep stirring until just incorporated.

Spread the batter into the already prepared pan & bake until the edges turn light brown, for 20 to 22 minutes. Don't over bake the bars or else they would become dry. Let them completely cool.

Now, blend butter & cream cheese until fluffy. Add confectioners' sugar & orange extract; beat until frosting is fluffy & spreadable (if required, feel free to add 1 teaspoon of milk). Spread it evenly over the cooled bars.

Remove the rind from an orange using a zester; sprinkle the zest on top of the frosted bars. Coarsely chop approximately 1/3 cup of the Craisins & then sprinkle on top of the frosted bars.

Now, in a glass measuring cup; mix oil & white chocolate. Microwave for a minute until melted; stirring after every 15 seconds. Whisk or use a fork to drizzle the melted white chocolate across the bars.

Before slicing into pieces, let it rest for an hour and let the white chocolate to completely set.

Nutrition: Calories: 156 kcal, Protein: 1.58 g, Fat: 7.4 g, Carbohydrates: 21.24 g

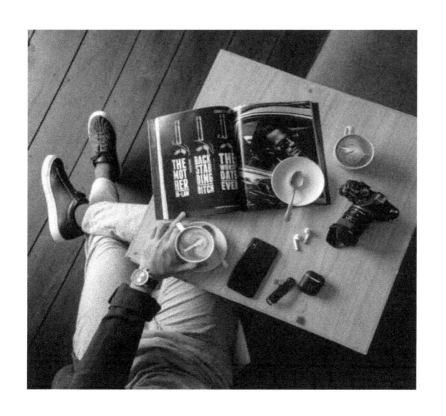

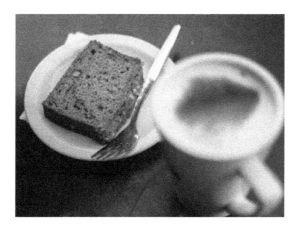

Soups and Side Dishes

Copycat Olive Garden's Creamy Zuppa Toscana

Preparation Time: 15 minutes

Cooking Time: 50 minutes

Servings: 4

Ingredients:

2 cups sweet yellow onion, quartered and sliced

½ cup sweet cream butter

½ teaspoon salt

1 tablespoon flour

4 cups beef stock

1 tablespoon fresh thyme

1 teaspoon coarse ground black pepper

4 baguette slices, approximately ½-inch thick

8 slices Provolone cheese

Directions:

Melt the butter in a stock pot over medium heat.

Add the onions and salt, and sauté for 3 minutes or until translucent but not browned. Add the flour and stir.

Add the beef stock, increase the heat to medium-high, and bring to a boil. Let boil for 1 minute.

Reduce the heat to low, season with thyme and black pepper. Cover and let simmer for 25-30 minutes.

While the soup is simmering, toast the baguette slices to a medium golden brown. Make sure each slice will fit comfortably in your soup bowl.

Preheat the broiler.

When the soup is done simmering, ladle it into oven proof serving bowls.

Top each bowl with a toasted baguette slice and 2 slices of Provolone cheese. Place under the broiler for 1-2 minutes, or until the cheese is well melted and lightly caramelized.

Remove from the broiler carefully and serve immediately

Nutrition: Calories: 420, Fat: 29 g, Carbs: 21 g, Protein: 19 g, Sodium: 2120 mg

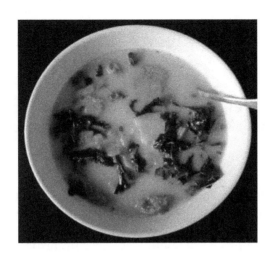

Red Lobster's Clam Chowder

Preparation Time: 20 minutes

Cooking Time: 30 minutes

Servings: 8

Ingredients:

2 tablespoons butter

1 cup onion, diced

½ cup leek, white part, thinly sliced

¼ teaspoon garlic, minced

½ cup celery, diced

2 tablespoons flour

4 cups milk

1 cup clams with juice, diced

1 cup potato, diced

1 tablespoon salt

¼ teaspoon white pepper

1 teaspoon dried thyme

½ cup heavy cream

Saltine crackers for serving

Directions:

In a pot, sauté the onion, leek, garlic, and celery in butter over medium heat.

After 3 minutes, remove the vegetables from the heat and add the flour.

Whisk in the milk and clam juice.

Return the mixture to the heat and bring it to a boil.

Add the potatoes, salt, pepper, and thyme, then lower the heat to let the mixture simmer. Continue mixing for another 10 minutes while the soup is simmering.

Add in the clams and let the mixture simmer for 5 to 8 minutes, or until the clams are cooked.

Add the heavy cream and cook for a few more minutes.

Transfer the soup to a bowl and serve with saltine crackers.

Nutrition: Calories: 436.1, Fat: 26.5 g, Carbs: 30.1 g, Protein: 20.3 g, Sodium: 1987 mg

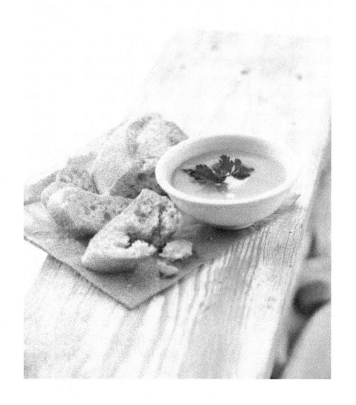

Carrabba's Mama Mandola Sicilian Chicken Soup

Preparation Time: 15 minutes

Cooking Time: 8 hours

Servings: 10

Ingredients:

4 carrots, peeled, diced

4 stalks celery, diced

1 green bell pepper, cored, diced

2 medium white potatoes, diced

1 white onion, diced

3 cloves garlic, minced

1 can (14.5 ounces) tomatoes, diced, with juice

1 tablespoon fresh parsley

1 teaspoon Italian seasoning

½ teaspoon white pepper

Dash of crushed red pepper flakes, to taste

2 boneless skinless chicken breasts, shredded

2 32-ounces containers chicken stock

1 ½ teaspoons salt

1 pound Ditalini pasta

Directions:

Dice and chop the vegetables as instructed.

Place them in a slow cooker and sprinkle with the parsley, seasoning, and white and red pepper. Mix everything together.

Add the shredded chicken and stock and mix again.

Cover the mixture and cook it for 8 hours on low heat.

When the soup is almost ready, bring a salt-and-water mixture to a boil to cook the pasta.

Add the cooked pasta to the soup and continue cooking for 5 minutes and serve.

Nutrition: Calories: 320, Fat: 0 g, Carbs: 57 g, Protein: 13 g, Sodium: 525.3 mg

Denny's Vegetable and Beef Barley Soup

Preparation Time: 10 minutes

Cooking Time: 40 minutes

Servings: 4

Ingredients:

½ pound ground beef

16 ounces frozen mixed vegetables

1 can (14.5 ounces) tomatoes, diced, with juice

¼ cup barley

32-ounce beef broth

Salt and pepper

Directions:

Place the ground beef in a pot and cook until brown.

Add in the vegetables, tomatoes, barley, and broth, and bring the entire mixture to a simmer.

Add salt and pepper for seasoning and leave the mixture to simmer for at least 40 minutes.

Ladle the soup into bowls and serve. The longer you leave the soup to simmer, the better it will taste.

Nutrition: Calories: 244.5, Fat: 11.4 g, Carbs: 17.1 g

Protein: 20 g, Sodium: 1818.2 mg

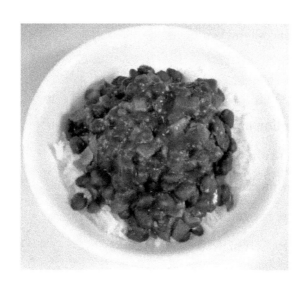

Outback's Walkabout Soup

Preparation Time: 10 minutes

Cooking Time: 45 minutes

Servings: 4

Ingredients:

Thick white Sauce:

3 tablespoons butter

3 tablespoons flour

¼ teaspoon salt

1½ cups whole milk

Soup:

2 cups yellow sweet onions, thinly sliced

3 tablespoons butter

1 can (14.5 ounces) chicken broth

½ teaspoon salt

¼ teaspoon fresh ground black pepper

2 chicken bouillon cubes

¼ cup Velveeta cubes, diced, packed

1½–1¾ cups white sauce (recipe above)

Cheddar cheese for garnish, shredded

Crusty bread for serving

Directions:

Make the thick white sauce first. Make a roux by cooking melted butter and flour over medium heat. Slowly pour the milk onto the roux, a little at a time, while constantly stirring the mixture. When the mixture reaches a pudding-like consistency, remove it from heat and set aside.

In a soup pot, sauté the onions in the butter over medium heat until they become translucent.

Add the rest of the ingredients, except the cheese and white sauce, to the pot and mix everything together.

When the mixture has heated up completely, add the cheese and white sauce. Bring the entire mixture to a simmer on medium-low heat. Continuously stir the soup until everything is completely mixed together.

When the cheese has melted, turn the heat lower and continue to cook the soup for another 30 to 45 minutes.

Ladle the soup into bowls and garnish with cheese. Serve with a side of bread.

Nutrition: Calories: 329, Fat: 25 g, Carbs: 17 g, Protein: 6 g, Sodium: 1061 mg

Wolfgang Puck's Butternut Squash Soup

Preparation Time: 25 minutes

Cooking Time: 1 hour and 15 minutes

Servings: 2 quarts

Ingredients:

Soup:

3¾ pounds butternut squash

1¾ pounds acorn squash

6 tablespoons unsalted butter, divided

1 onion, finely diced

½ teaspoon kosher salt

⅛ teaspoon fresh white pepper

¼ teaspoon ground nutmeg

¼ teaspoon ginger, ground

⅛ teaspoon ground cardamom

4 cups chicken or vegetable stock, warmed

½ cup crème fraiche

1 tablespoon thinly sliced fresh chives

Roasted Red Pepper Coulis:

2 red bell peppers

¼ cup chicken broth

Salt and pepper

Directions:

Preheat the oven to 350°F. Melt 2 tablespoons of the butter and season with salt, pepper, and nutmeg.

Prepare the squashes by cutting them in half, removing the seeds, and brushing the cut sides with the seasoned butter.

Line the squashes, cut-side down, on a baking pan. Bake for an hour.

When the squashes are soft, scoop them out into a bowl and purée. Set the squash purée aside.

Sauté the onions in 4 tablespoons of butter over low heat. Do not let them turn brown.

When the onions become translucent, add in the squash purée and allow the mixture to continue cooking. Make sure that the mixture does not simmer or boil.

When the mixture is heated through, add in the ginger and cardamom, then pour in the stock.

Without increasing the heat, bring the mixture to a boil. Allow the mixture to cook for 20 minutes while stirring occasionally.

Meanwhile, make the red pepper coulis:

a)   Roast the bell peppers over flame until the skin is charred or in oven under the broiler. Let the pepper cool down.

b)   Peel of the skin of the peppers and then purée the flesh while slowly pouring in the chicken broth.

c)   Season with salt and pepper.

d)   Transfer to a sauce bottle and set aside.

When the mixture has cooked through, add in the crème fraiche and chives.

When the flavors have mixed, remove the rosemary sprig and season the soup to your liking.

Transfer the mixture to a bowl and squeeze the red pepper coulis over the soup, creating swirls before serving.

Nutrition: Calories: 1293.8, Fat: 64.3 g, Carbs: 172.8 g, Protein: 27.9 g, Sodium: 1296.3 mg

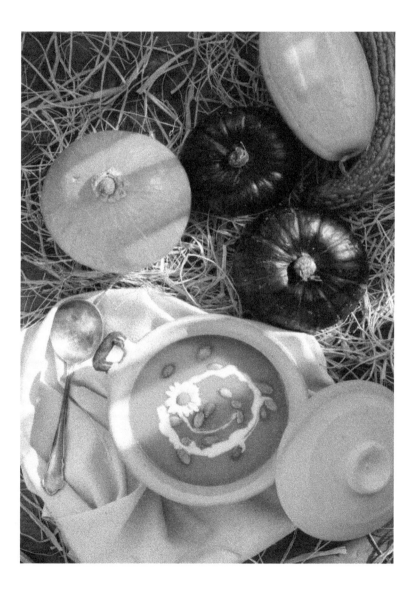

Frijoles Negros (Cuban Black Beans)

Preparation Time: 30 minutes

Cooking Time: 1 hour

Servings: 8

Ingredients:

450 grams of black beans

10 cups of Water (2400 milliliters)

6 tablespoons olive oil

1 unit large onion

5 cloves of garlic

¼ tablespoon oregano dessert

1 bay leaf

¼ tablespoon ground cumin dessert

1 pinch of salt

1 pinch of pepper

1 tablespoon vinegar

1 tablespoon dry wine

1 tablespoon of sugar

1 unit large green chili pepper

Directions:

To start with our recipe for Cuban beans, the first thing we are going to do is to wash the beans well and soak them with water and a bay leaf. Ideally, leave them overnight so that they inflate and you can cook them better.

The next day, take a pot with enough capacity, pour the beans in it with the water and the bay leaf and cook them for approximately 45 minutes, until they are soft.

When they are ready, drain them and prepare the black bean stir - fry. To do this, take a deep pan and heat the olive oil. Once hot, add the finely chopped onion and chili, or crushed if desired, and crushed garlic. Remove it with a wooden spoon and fry it.

Of the already soft beans, reserve a cup for later, the rest add it to the frypan, with the blade included. Remove everything, add salt and pepper to taste, oregano, cumin, and sugar and simmer for a few minutes. Do not stop stirring to prevent black beans from sticking and burning.

Then, mash the beans you reserved in the cup, add them to the rest and simmer them for half an hour and with the pan covered.

After the time, add the dry wine and the vinegar, stir it well and let it rest with the fire for at least 10 minutes. When they are ready to add two tablespoons of olive oil, integrate it and serve the black beans to the Cuban accompanied by white rice.

Nutrition: Calories: 172kcal, Carbohydrates: 18 g, Fat: 9 g, Saturated fat: 5 g, Potassium: 369 mg, Protein: 6 g, Sodium: 294 mg, Fiber: 7 g, Sugar: 1 g, Vitamin A: 111IU, Vitamin C: 9 mg, Calcium: 23 mg, Iron: 1 mg

Oven Roasted Brussel Sprouts

Preparation Time: 50 minutes

Cooking Time: 30 minutes

Servings: 6

Ingredients:

500 grams of Brussels sprouts

3 tablespoons olive oil

2 tablespoons balsamic vinegar of Modena

2 tablespoons honey (or agave syrup or another sugar-free substitute)

Salt to taste Ground black pepper to taste

Directions:

Wash the cabbages and remove the top layers when necessary. We split them in half. Place the cabbage in a bowl and add the olive oil. We mix well.

Then, add the vinegar, honey or syrup and season to taste. We mix well.

Place the mixture on a baking sheet lined with vegetable paper with the inside of the cabbages facing up, and cook the Brussels sprouts in the oven and hot at 200°C at half-height about 20 minutes until golden brown and tender.

You will see how rich the roasted Brussels sprouts are left with that bittersweet mixture and the golden-brown of the oven. I can't think of a better way to enjoy this vegetable. Really, superior!

Nutrition: Calories: 357kcal, Carbohydrates: 42 g, Fat: 21 g, Saturated fat: 12 g, Carbs: 31 g, Protein: 5 g, Sodium: 334 mg, Sugar: 31 g, Fiber: 3 g, Vitamin A: 4598IU, Potassium: 503 mg, Vitamin C: 97 mg, Calcium: 116 mg, Iron: 2 mg

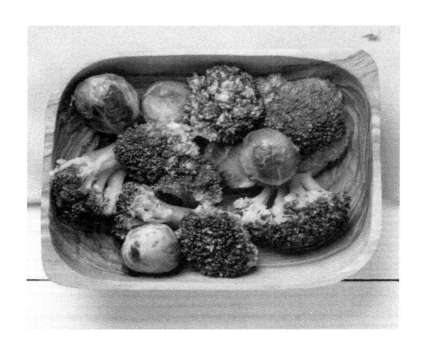

Garlic Green Beans

Preparation Time: 20 minutes

Cooking Time: 30 minutes

Servings: 10

Ingredients:

800 g of fresh green beans

2 cloves of garlic

1 tablet of vegetable broth

1 teaspoon chopped thyme

1 lemon

2 tablespoons olive oil

Salt

Directions:

Cut the ends of the beans, remove the strands and chop them. Peel and crush the garlic cloves together with the thyme in a mortar.

Put the oil in a pan and sauté the beans 3 or 4 minutes, add the mashed garlic and saute 3 more minutes over low heat, without letting the garlic burn.

Add water just to cover, pour the crumbled broth and salt to taste. Cook until the beans are tender (about 15-20 minutes), drain them and water them with the lemon juice.

Nutrition: Calories: 175kcal, Carbohydrates: 17 g, Saturated fat: 7 g, Cholesterol: 30 mg, Potassium: 479 mg, Fat: 12 g, Sugar: 7 g, Fiber: 6 g, Protein: 4 g, Sodium: 114 mg, Vitamin A: 1915IU, Vitamin C: 29 mg, Calcium: 89 mg, Iron: 2 mg

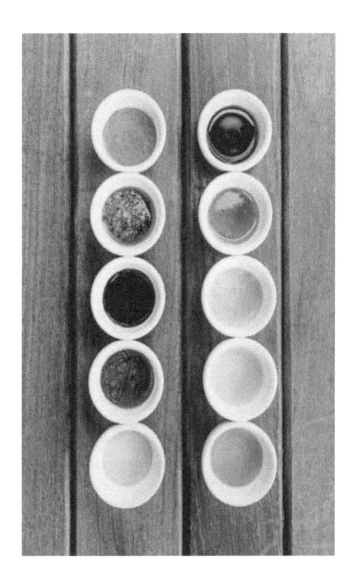

Souces and Dressing

Kraft Thousand Island dressing

Preparation Time: 5 minutes

Cooking Time: none

Servings: 16

Ingredients:

1 cup mayonnaise

¼ cup ketchup

2 tablespoons white vinegar

4 teaspoons white sugar

2 teaspoons sweet pickle relish, minced

2 teaspoons white onion, finely chopped or minced

¼ teaspoon sea salt

¼ teaspoon black pepper

Directions:

Take a large bowl and combine all the ingredients in it.

Mix well.

Serve.

Enjoy.

Nutrition: Calories: 67, Fat: 4.9 g, Carbs: 6 g, Protein: 2 g, Sodium: 167 mg

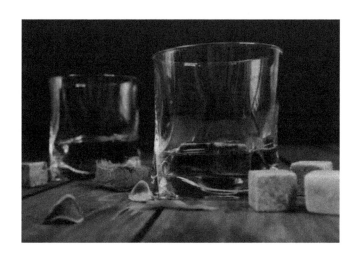

Newman Own's Creamy Caesar Salad Dressing

Preparation Time: 5 minutes

Cooking Time: 0

Servings: 10

Ingredients:

2 cups mayonnaise

6 tablespoons white vinegar, distilled

¼ cup Parmesan cheese, grated

4 teaspoons Worcestershire sauce

1 teaspoon lime juice

1 teaspoon dry mustard, ground   ⅓ teaspoon salt, or to taste

½ teaspoon garlic powder   ½ teaspoon onion powder

½ teaspoon black pepper, freshly ground

1 pinch basil, dried

1 pinch oregano, dried

Directions:

Take an electric mixer and blend all the ingredients until smooth.

Chill the prepared dressing for a few hours before severing.

Enjoy.

Nutrition: Calories: 215, Fat: 17.4 g, Carbs: 13.3 g, Protein: 2.3 g, Sodium: 540 mg

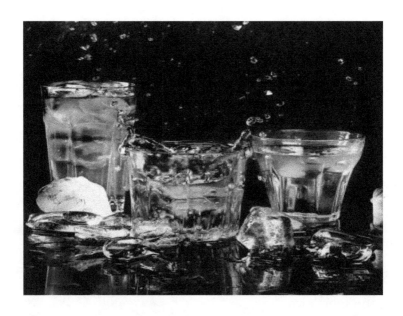

Bull's Eye Original BBQ Sauce

Preparation Time: 20 minutes

Cooking Time: 15 minutes

Servings: yield 2 cups

Ingredients:

1½ cups tomato ketchup

½ cup Worcestershire sauce

5 tablespoons butter, melted

¼ cup white vinegar

1 tablespoon yellow mustard

¼ cup onions, finely minced

2 tablespoons hickory liquid smoke

½ teaspoon Tabasco sauce

1 cup sugar, brown

1 tablespoon white sugar

Salt, to taste

Directions:

Combine the ingredients in a saucepan and heat it over medium heat.

Simmer the ingredients for 15 minutes, stirring occasionally.

Turn off the heat and let the sauce get cold.

The sauce is ready.

Nutrition: Calories: 112, Fat: 3.7 g, Carbs: 20.5 g, Protein: 0.5 g, Sodium: 386 mg

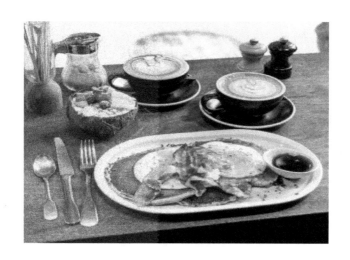

Kraft Miracle Whip

Preparation Time: 20 minutes

Cooking Time: 15 minutes

Servings: 1 ½ cups

Ingredients:

4 egg yolks

⅓ teaspoon salt

2 tablespoons powdered sugar

6 tablespoons lemon juice

2 cups oil

2 tablespoons cornstarch

2 teaspoons dry mustard

1 cup boiling water

¼ cup vinegar

Table salt, to taste

Directions:

Take a blender and add egg yolks along with salt, sugar, and half of lemon juice.

Blend for few seconds until combined.

While the blender is running, start adding the oil, a few drops at a time.

Add the remaining lemon juice.

Turn off the blender.

In a bowl, mix together cornstarch, water, mustard, and vinegar.

Mix until a smooth paste is formed.

Pour the bowl ingredients into a pan.

Cook on low heat until thickened.

Slowly add this cooked mixture into the blender.

Turn on the blender and combine all the ingredients well.

Transfer to a jar and let cool in the refrigerator.

Nutrition: Calories: 432, Fat: 49. 1g, Carbs: 0. 9 g, Protein: 4.3 g, Sodium: 564 mg

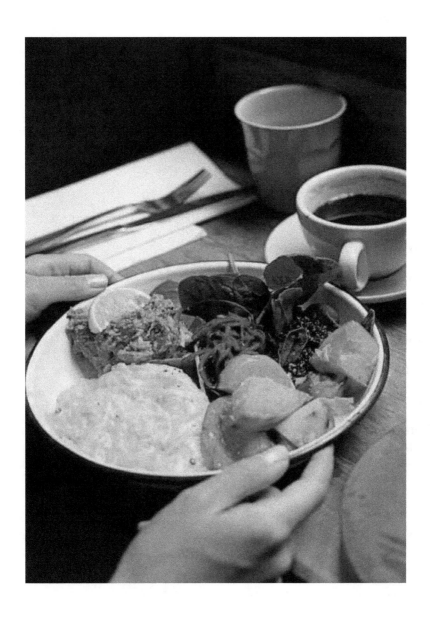

Hellman's Mayonnaise

Preparation Time: 15 minutes

Cooking Time: none

Servings: 1 cup

Ingredients:

3 large egg yolks

1 teaspoon dry mustard

1 teaspoon salt

½ teaspoon cayenne pepper

1½ cups canola oil

4-6 tablespoons lemon juice

Directions:

Add mustard and egg yolks into a blender and pulse until combined.

While the blender is blending set the speed to low and start adding the oil very slowly.

Stop the blender and scrape down the mayonnaise.

Add the lemon juice and remaining oil.

Keep on blending until combined.

At the end add salt and cayenne pepper.

Mix and serve.

Nutrition: Calories: 362, Fat: 39.1, Carbs: 0.7 g, Protein: 3.4 g, Sodium: 425 mg

Heinz Ketchup

Preparation Time: 25 minutes

Cooking Time: 20 minutes

Servings: yield about 1 and ½ cups

Ingredients:

1 cup tomato paste

⅓ cup light corn syrup

½ cup white vinegar

⅓ cup water

2 tablespoons sugar

Salt, to taste

⅓ teaspoon onion powder

¼ teaspoon garlic powder

Directions:

Combine all the ingredients in a saucepan.

Turn on the heat and let the liquid simmer for 20 minutes.

Turn off the heat and let the mixture cool down.

Store in airtight glass jar or serve with French fries.

Nutrition: Calories: 78, Fat: 0.2 g, Carbs: 19.3 g

Protein: 1.4 g, Sodium: 53 mg

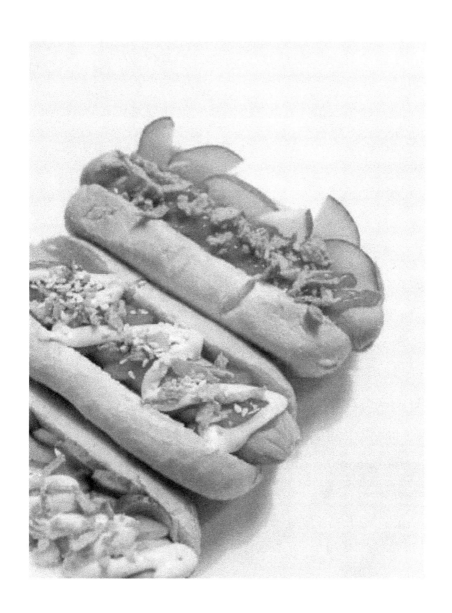

395

Hidden Valley Original Ranch Dressing

Preparation Time: 10 minutes

Cooking Time: none

Servings: 6

Ingredients:

1 cup mayonnaise

1 cup buttermilk

1 teaspoon parsley flakes, dried

½ teaspoon black pepper, ground

⅓ teaspoon sea salt

¼ teaspoon garlic powder

¼ teaspoon onion powder

2 pinches of thyme, dried

Directions:

Take a blender and combine all the ingredients in it.

Pulse until smooth.

Transfer to a glass jar and chill in refrigerator before serving.

Nutrition: Calories: 170, Fat: 13.5 g, Carbs: 11.7 g, Protein: 1.8 g, Sodium: 427 mg

Carrabba's Bread Dipping Blend

Preparation Time: 10 minutes

Cooking Time: 10 minutes

Servings: 8

Ingredients:

1 tablespoon red pepper, crushed

1 ½ teaspoon garlic powder

1 tablespoon dried parsley

½ teaspoon dried rosemary

1 tablespoon dried basil

1 ½ teaspoon onion powder

1 tablespoon dried oregano

3 garlic cloves, fresh, crushed

Extra virgin olive oil, as required

1 tablespoon freshly cracked black pepper

1 ½ teaspoon coarse sea salt

Directions:

Combine black pepper together with the parsley, crushed red pepper, basil, oregano, onion powder, garlic powder, rosemary, crush garlic and sea salt; mix well.

Place the dry spice mixture in a large-sized shallow plate & drizzle with the extra virgin olive oil. Mix well & serve.

Nutrition: Calories: 243, Fat: 89.3 g, Carbs: 15.4 g, Protein: 24.8 g, Sodium: 1687 mg

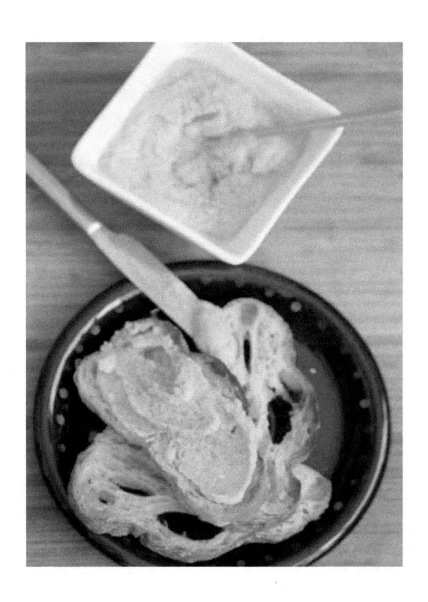

California Pizza Kitchen Tuscan Hummus

Preparation Time: 30 minutes

Cooking Time: 30 minutes

Servings: 6

Ingredients:

10 garlic cloves

½ cup tahini or sesame paste

2 cans great northern or cannellini beans, drained (15-ounce size)

1/8 teaspoon ground coriander

1 tablespoon plus ½ teaspoon soy sauce

¼ cup lemon juice, freshly squeezed

1 ½ teaspoon cumin

½ teaspoon cayenne pepper

2 tablespoons fresh Italian parsley, minced

1 ½ teaspoon salt

¼ cup cold water, if required

For California Pizza Kitchen Checca:

2 pounds Roma tomatoes, cut into ½" dice

1 tablespoon fresh basil, minced

½ cup extra-virgin olive oil

1 tablespoon garlic, minced

2 teaspoons salt

Directions:

Process the garlic cloves in a food processor attached with a steel blade until minced finely, stopping & scrapping the sides of the work bowl occasionally, as required.

Add in the cannellini beans & pulse again until coarsely chopped. Then, with the machine still running on low speed, slowly pour the sesame paste through the feed tube & puree. Don't just turn off the motor; pour in the soy sauce, olive oil and lemon juice through the feed tube (stopping & scrapping down the sides, as required).

Stop; remove the lid & add cumin, cayenne, coriander and salt. Process again until blended thoroughly. Feel free to add ¼ to ½ cup of cold water to the mix and pulse, if the puree seems to be too thick for spreading or dipping. Transfer the puree to a large bowl & cover with a plastic wrap; let refrigerate until chill.

In the meantime; preheat your oven to 250 F in advance.

Place the pita breads in the preheated oven & heat for a couple of minutes, until thoroughly warmed.

Carefully remove the breads & cut into desired wedges. Place the chilled hummus in a serving bowl or plate & arrange the tomato Checca over the top. Garnish with the freshly chopped parsley & surround with the pita triangles. Serve immediately and enjoy.

For California Pizza Kitchen Checca:

Toss the entire Checca ingredients together in a large-sized mixing bowl; continue to toss until thoroughly mixed. Using a plastic wrap; cover & refrigerate until ready to use.

Nutrition: Calories: 134, Fat: 67 g, Carbs: 52. 5 g, Protein: 64 g, Sodium: 1254 mg

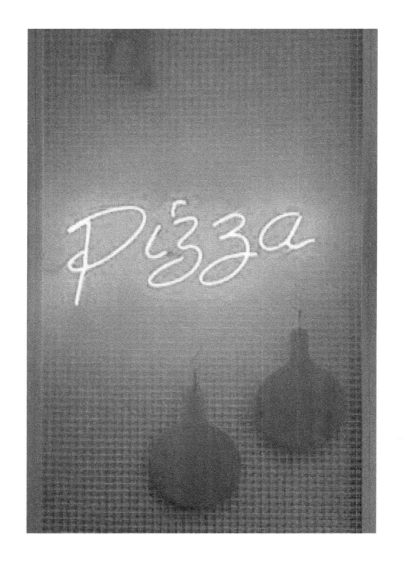

Pizza

Cheddar's Santa Fe Spinach Dip

Preparation Time: 5 minutes

Cooking Time: 20 minutes

Servings: 6

Ingredients:

2 packages chopped spinach, frozen (10 ounces each)

1 cup heavy whipping cream

2.4 ounces Monterey jack cheese; cut it into 3 equal 2" long blocks

1 package cream cheese (8 oz)

2.4 ounces pepper jack cheese; cut it into 3 equal 2" long blocks

½ cup Sour Cream

2.4 ounces White American Cheese; cut it into 3 equal 2" long blocks

½ to 1 teaspoon salsa seasoning

2 teaspoon Alfredo sauce

1 cup mozzarella cheese

Pepper & salt to taste

Directions:

Over low-heat in a large pan; heat the chopped spinach until all the moisture is cooked out, for a couple of minutes, stirring frequently.

In the meantime, over moderate heat in a large pot; add in the cream cheese & 1 cup of heavy whipping cream; cook until the cheese is completely melted; ensure that you don't really bring it to a boil. Feel free to decrease the heat, if it starts to boil.

Once done; work in batches and start adding the Pepper Jack, Monterey Jack & White American cheeses. Continue to stir the ingredients & don't let it come to a boil.

Lastly add in the Mozzarella cheese and continue to cook.

Add 2 teaspoons of the Alfredo sauce and then add in the cooked spinach.

Add ½ cup of the sour cream; continue to mix until combined well.

Add salsa seasoning, pepper & salt to taste; stir well

Serve immediately with some tortilla chips & enjoy!

Nutrition: Calories: 177, Fat: 12. 6 g, Carbs: 35. 8 g, Protein: 37. 8 g, Sodium: 677 mg

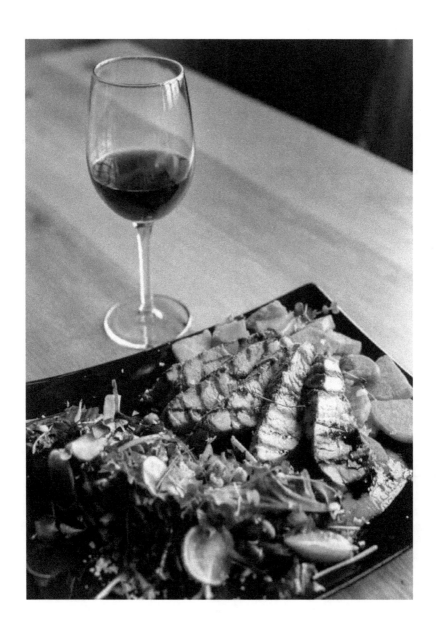

Olive Garden Hot Artichoke Spinach Dip

Preparation Time: 30 minutes

Cooking Time: 30 minutes

Servings: 4

Ingredients:

½ cup chopped spinach, frozen, thawed & well drained

1 package (8-ounce size) cream cheese, at room temperature

¼ cup each of Mozzarella cheese, Romano cheese & Parmesan cheese, shredded

1 garlic clove, minced finely

¼ cup mayonnaise

1 can artichoke hearts, drained & coarsely chopped (14 ounce)

½ teaspoon dried basil

¼ teaspoon garlic salt

Directions:

Lightly grease a large-sized glass pie plate and preheat your oven to 350 F in advance.

Beat the cream cheese together with Romano cheese, Parmesan cheese, mayonnaise, basil, garlic & garlic salt in a large-sized mixing bowl; beat well.

Stir in the spinach and artichoke hearts until mixed well.

When ready, spoon the dip into the greased pie plate & evenly sprinkle the top with the Mozzarella cheese.

Place the dip in the oven and bake until the Mozzarella cheese is completely melted & turns lightly browned, for 25 minutes, at 350 F.

Remove the dip from oven & serve hot with some crackers or toasted bread slices for dipping.

Nutrition: Calories: 143, Fat: 6.9 g, Carbs: 65 g, Protein: 26 g, Sodium: 376 mg

Olive Garden Spinach-Artichoke Dip

Preparation Time: 3 minutes

Cooking Time: 35 minutes

Servings: 10

Ingredients:

1 can artichoke hearts, drained, coarsely chopped (14 ounce)

¼ cup mayonnaise

1 package light cream cheese (8 ounce); at room temperature

¼ cup parmesan cheese

½ cup chopped spinach, frozen

¼ cup Romano cheese

1 garlic clove, minced finely

¼ cup mozzarella cheese, grated

½ teaspoon dry basil or 1 tablespoon fresh

¼ teaspoon garlic salt

Pepper & salt to taste

Directions:

Combine cream cheese together with mayonnaise Romano cheese, Parmesan, basil, garlic & garlic salt; mix until combined well.

Add in the drained spinach and artichoke hearts; mix until well blended.

Spray a pie pan with Pam and then pour in the dip; top with the Mozzarella cheese.

Bake until the top is browned, for 25 minutes, at 350 F.

Serve with Italian or French toasted bread, thinly sliced.

Nutrition: Calories: 563, Fat: 14. 3 g, Carbs: 76. 8 g, Protein: 54. 8 g, Sodium: 1434. 7 mg

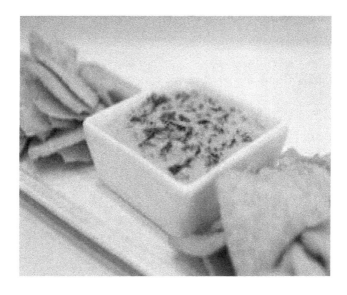

Houston's Chicago Style Spinach Dip

Preparation Time: 5 minutes

Cooking Time: 15 minutes

Servings: 10

Ingredients:

⅓ cup sour cream

2 bags of fresh Spinach (1 pound each)

⅔ cup fresh parmesan cheese, grated

1 can Artichoke Hearts, coarsely diced

1/8 pound butter

2 tablespoons onions, minced

½ cup Monterrey Jack Cheese, grated

1 teaspoon fresh garlic, minced

½ teaspoon Tabasco sauce or to taste

1 pint heavy whipping cream

¼ cup flour

2 teaspoons lemon juice, freshly squeezed

½ teaspoon salt

Directions:

Steam the spinach; strain & using a cheese cloth; squeeze the water out. Finely chop & set aside until ready to use.

Now, over moderate heat in a heavy saucepan; heat the butter until completely melted.

Add in the onions and garlic; sauté for 3 to 5 minutes.

Make a roux by adding the flour. Give everything a good stir & cook for a minute.

Slowly add in the heavy cream, stirring with a whisk to prevent lumping. The mixture would thicken at the boiling point.

When done, immediately add in the Tabasco, lemon juice, Parmesan cheese and salt.

Immediately remove the pan from heat & let stand at room temperature for 5 minutes and then stir in the sour cream.

Fold in the diced artichoke hearts, Jack cheese and dry & chopped spinach. Stir well until the cheese is completely melted.

Serve immediately and enjoy.

Nutrition: Calories: 476. 6, Fat: 53. 6 g, Carbs: 78. 7 g, Protein: 27. 7 g, Sodium: 2868 mg

Ruby Tuesday Queso Dip

Preparation Time: 10 minutes

Cooking Time: 10 minutes

Servings: 6

Ingredients:

1 box chopped spinach, frozen, thawed & squeeze out any excess water (approximately 10 oz)

1 jar of Taco Bell salsa & queso (approximately 14 oz)

Directions:

Mix the entire ingredients together in a microwave-safe bowl. Heat in 1-minute intervals on high-power, stirring frequently. Continue to heat in the microwave until heated through. Serve with your favorite tortilla chips and enjoy.

Nutrition: Calories: 257, Fat: 47.7 g, Carbs: 86. 6 g, Protein: 28. 7 g, Sodium: 2498 mg

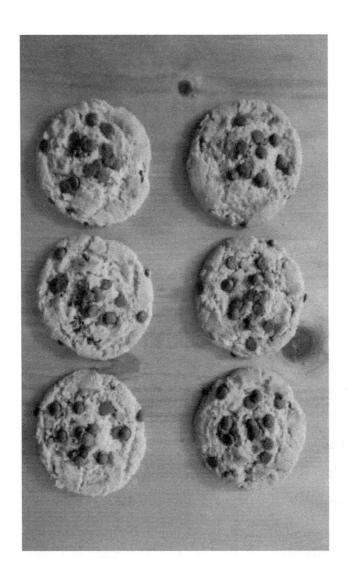

Desserts

Panera Bread's Chocolate Chip Cookies

Preparation Time: 15 minutes

Cooking Time: 15 minutes

Servings: 12

Ingredients:

2½ sticks unsalted butter

1¼ cup dark brown sugar

¼ cup granulated sugar

2 teaspoons vanilla extract

2 eggs

3½ cups all-purpose flour

1 tablespoon cornstarch

1 teaspoon baking soda

1 teaspoon salt

1 bag (12 ounces) mini semisweet chocolate chips

Directions:

Cream the butter and sugars using a whisk or a hand mixer.

Whip in the vanilla extract and eggs and set the wet mixture aside.

In a different bowl, mix together the flour, cornstarch, baking soda, and salt.

Pour the dry mixture into the wet mixture a little at a time, folding with a spatula. Add in the chocolate chips and continue folding.

Roll the cookie dough into balls and place them on a baking sheet. Place the baking sheet in the freezer for 15 minutes.

Preheat the oven to 350°F while waiting for the cookies to harden.

Transfer the cookies from the freezer to the oven immediately and bake for 15 minutes.

Nutrition: Calories: 440, Fat: 23 g, Carbs: 59 g, Protein: 4 g, Sodium: 240 mg

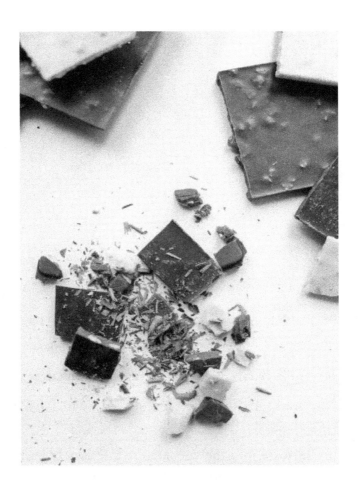

Applebee's Maple Butter Blondie

Preparation Time: 10 minutes

Cooking Time: 25 minutes

Servings: 6

Ingredients:

⅓ cup butter, melted

1 cup brown sugar, packed

1 egg, beaten

1 tablespoon vanilla extract

1 cup all-purpose flour

½ teaspoon baking powder

⅛ teaspoon baking soda

⅛ teaspoon salt

½ cup white chocolate chips

½ cup walnuts or pecans, chopped

Maple Cream Sauce:

½ cup maple syrup

¼ cup butter

½ cup brown sugar

8 ounces cream cheese, softened

Walnuts for garnish, chopped; optional

Vanilla ice cream for serving

Directions:

Prepare your materials by:

a)   Preheating the oven to 350°F; and

b)   Greasing an 8×8 baking pan.

Dissolve the sugar in the melted butter. Whip in the egg and the vanilla and set the mixture aside.

In another bowl, mix together the flour, baking powder and soda, and salt.

Slowly pour the dry mixture into the butter mixture and mix thoroughly.

Make sure the mixture is at room temperature before folding in the nuts and chocolate chips.

Transfer the mixture into the baking pan and bake for 20 to 25 minutes.

While waiting for the blondies to bake, combine the syrup and butter over low heat. When the butter has melted, mix in the sugar and cream cheese. Take the mixture off the heat when the cream cheese has melted, and set aside.

Let the blondies cool a little and then cut them into rectangles. Serve with the syrup, top with walnuts and vanilla ice cream, if desired, and serve.

Nutrition: Calories: 1000, Fat: 54 g, Carbs: 117 g, Protein: 13 g, Sodium: 620 mg

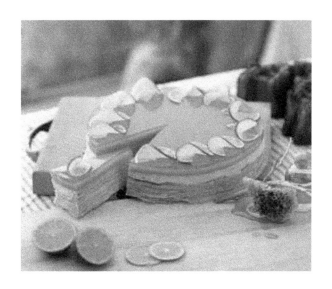

Tommy Bahama's Key Lime Pie

Preparation Time: 40 minutes

Cooking Time: 50 minutes

Servings: 2

Ingredients:

Pie:

10-inch graham cracker crust

1 egg white

2½ cups sweetened condensed milk

¾ cup pasteurized egg yolk

1 cup lime juice

1 lime, zest

1 lime, sliced into 8

White Chocolate Mousse Whipped Cream:

8 fluid ounces heavy cream

3 tablespoons powdered sugar

¼ teaspoon pure vanilla extract

½ tablespoon white chocolate mousse instant mix

Directions:

Preheat the oven to 350°F while brushing the graham cracker crust with the egg white. Cover the crust completely before placing it in the oven to bake for 5 minutes.

Whip the egg yolk and condensed milk together until they are blended completely. Add the lime juice and zest to the mixture and continue whipping until the mixture is smooth.

If you haven't yet, remove the crust from the oven and let it cool. When the crust has cooled, add in the egg mixture and bake at 250°F for 25 to 30 minutes.

When the pie is cooked, place it on a cooling rack to cool. Then place it in the refrigerator for at least two hours.

While waiting for the pie to cool, beat the first three whipped cream ingredients for two minutes (if using a hand mixer). When the mixture is smooth, add in the chocolate mousse and beat to stiff peaks.

Remove the pie from the refrigerator, slice it into eight pieces, and garnish each with the white chocolate mousse whipped cream and a slice of lime. Serve.

Nutrition: Calories: 500, Fat: 9 g, Carbs: 26 g, Protein: 1 g, Sodium: 110 mg

Dairy Queen's Blizzard

Preparation Time: 5 minutes

Cooking Time: 0 minutes

Servings: 1

Ingredients:

1 candy bar, of your choice

¼ to ½ cup milk

2½ cups vanilla ice cream

1 teaspoon fudge sauce

Directions:

Place the candy bar of your choice into the freezer to harden it.

Break the candy bar into multiple tiny chunks and place all the ingredients into a blender.

Keep blending until the ice cream becomes thicker and everything is mixed completely.

Pour into a cup and consume.

Nutrition: Calories: 953, Fat: 51.6 g, Carbs: 108.8 g, Protein: 15.1 g, Sodium: 439.4 mg

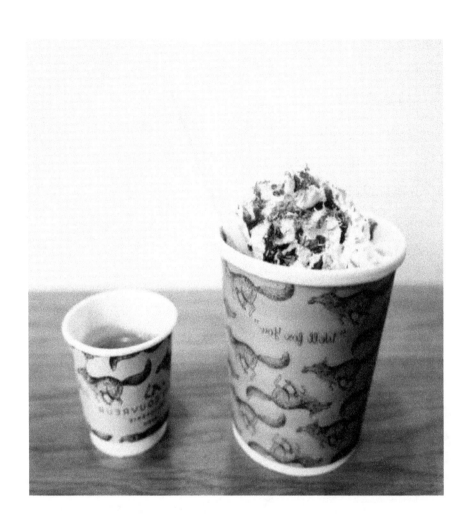

Olive Garden's Tiramisu

Preparation Time: 10 minutes

Cooking Time: 2 hours and 50 minutes

Servings: 9

Ingredients:

4 egg yolks

2 tablespoons milk

⅔ cup granulated sugar

2 cups mascarpone cheese

¼ teaspoon vanilla extract

1 cup heavy cream

½ cup cold espresso

¼ cup Kahlua

20–24 ladyfingers

2 teaspoons cocoa powder

Directions:

Bring water to a boil, then reduce the heat to maintain a simmer. Place a heatproof bowl over the water, making sure that the bowl does not touch the water.

In the heatproof bowl, whisk together the egg yolks, milk and sugar for about 8 to 10 minutes.

When the mixture has thickened, remove the bowl from heat and then whisk in the vanilla and mascarpone cheese until the mixture becomes smooth.

In another bowl, whisk the cream until soft peaks are formed.

Using a spatula, fold the whipped cream into the mascarpone mixture, making sure to retain the fluffiness of the whipped cream.

In another bowl, mix the espresso and Kahlua.

Dip the ladyfingers into the espresso mixture one by one. Dip only the bottom, and dip them quickly so as not to make them soggy.

Cover the bottom of an 8×8 pan with half of the dipped ladyfingers, cracking them if necessary.

Pour half of the mascarpone mixture over the ladyfingers.

Place another layer of ladyfingers over the mixture.

Pour the rest of the mixture over the second layer of ladyfingers and smooth out the top.

Dust some cocoa powder over the top and then place in the refrigerator.

Slice the cake and serve when set.

Nutrition: Calories: 288.6, Fat: 14 g, Carbs: 34.4 g, Protein: 4.4 g, Sodium: 53.6 mg

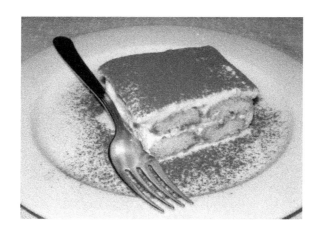

Cheesecake Factory's Oreo Cheesecake

Preparation Time: 25 minutes

Cooking Time: 1 hour

Servings: 10

Ingredients:

Crust:

1½ cups Oreo cookies, crushed

2 tablespoons butter, melted

Filling:

3 packages (8 ounces each) cream cheese, room temperature

1 cup sugar

5 large eggs, room temperature

2 teaspoons vanilla extract

¼ teaspoon salt

¼ cup all-purpose flour

1 container (8 ounces) sour cream, room temperature

14 Oreo cookies, divided

Directions:

To make the crust, crush whole Oreos in a blender or smash them with a rolling pin and mix them with the melted butter. Press the Oreo mixture to the bottom and sides of a 9-inch spring form pan.

Leave the crust to rest and preheat the oven to 325°F. Before starting to make the filling, make sure all of your ingredients are at room temperature.

Place the cream cheese in a medium-sized bowl and beat it with a hand mixer or a whisk until it is light and fluffy.

Beat in the sugar, mixing continuously so that the sugar is evenly distributed throughout the mixture.

Beat in the eggs, one at a time, and then add in the vanilla, salt, and flour. When the ingredients are all mixed together, add in the sour cream and 6 chopped Oreos.

Pour the filling onto the crust and then top with 8 whole Oreos.

Bake in the oven for an hour to an hour and 15 minutes. When the cake is done baking, leave it in the oven with the door open for an hour.

When it has cooled down, transfer the cake to the refrigerator. Leave it for a day or more before serving.

Nutrition: Calories: 1520, Fat: 55 g, Carbs: 175 g, Protein: 0 g, Sodium: 736 mg

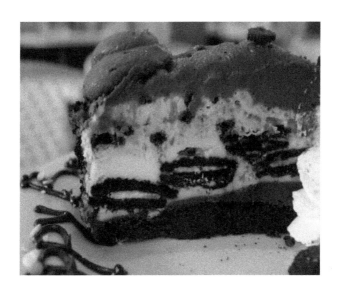

P.F. Chang's Ginger Panna Cotta

Preparation Time: 10 minutes

Cooking Time: 4 hours and 10 minutes

Servings: 3

Ingredients:

Panna Cotta:

¼ cup heavy cream

½ cup granulated sugar

1 tablespoon grated ginger

1½ tablespoons powdered gelatin

6 tablespoons warm water

Strawberry Sauce:

2 pounds ripe strawberries, hulled

½ cup granulated sugar

2 teaspoons cornstarch

½ lemon, juice

1 pinch salt

Directions:

Place the cream, sugar and ginger in a saucepan and cook over medium-low heat, until the sugar dissolves. Remove the mixture from heat and set aside.

In a medium-sized bowl, mix the water and the gelatin together. Set aside for a few minutes.

After the gelatin has rested, pour the sugar mixture into the medium-sized bowl and stir, removing all lumps.

Grease your ramekins and then transfer the mixture into the ramekins, leaving 2 inches of space at the top.

Place the ramekins in your refrigerator or freezer to let them set for at least 4 hours.

While the panna cottas are setting, make the strawberry sauce by cooking all the sauce ingredients in a medium-sized pan for 10 minutes. Stir the mixture occasionally, then remove from heat.

When the panna cottas are ready, flip over the containers onto a plate and allow the gelatin to stand. Drizzle with the strawberry sauce and serve.

Nutrition: Calories: 346, Fat: 30 g, Carbs: 16 g, Protein: 4 g, Sodium: 50 mg

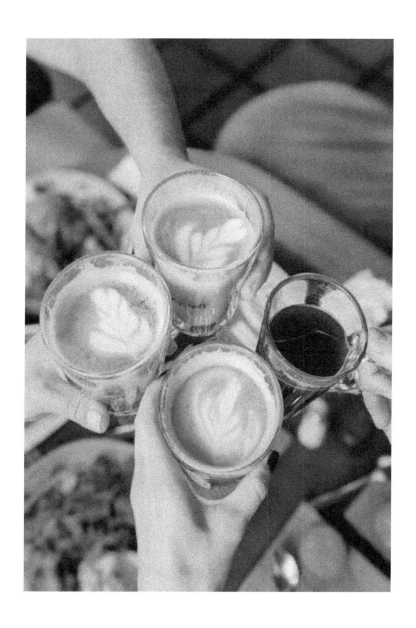

Conclusion

When preparing desserts at home, you can tweak the recipes as you wish. As you sample the recipes, you'll get to know the usual ingredients and techniques in making popular sweet treats. This could inspire you to create your very own recipes. You can substitute ingredients as your taste, health or pocket dictates. You can come up, perhaps, not with a dessert that's the perfect clone of a restaurant's recipe, but with one that's exactly the way you want it to be. Most of all, the recipes here are meant for you to experience the fulfillment of seeing the smiles on the people with whom you share your creations. Keep trying and having fun with these recipes and you'll soon be reaping your sweet rewards!

Reasons Copycat Recipes Are Better Than Eating at Restaurants

Imagine sitting at your favorite restaurant in the booth and your waitress has just placed your favorite hot piping dish before you. Smells so sweet! But it can be very expensive to eat out several times a week. What if you could have the exact recipe to make your favorite dish whenever you wish? What if you had over 100 home-made restaurant recipes to fix? Do the copycat recipes taste the real thing?

We are doing that, totally! Copycat recipes are constantly being tested to ensure that you create the restaurant's exact dishes. Expert chefs spend hours tailoring these recipes to get the perfect flavor. Such recipes are as close to the real thing as being in your own kitchen right at your favorite restaurant. How will you save money on these copycat recipes?

With these recipes the amount of money you'll save will be absolutely shocking. Imagine spending a night out at your favorite restaurant, for you and your significant other. You get an appetizer, 2 begins and a dessert is shared. You spent between $55 and $70 comfortably with beverages, food and a tip. You will probably spend about a third of that on producing these same recipes at home without losing any taste. So you could use the copycat recipes to prepare 3 different meals at home for what it would cost you to eat out once. So where are these recipes you looking at?

That's the copycat recipe's great thing. You won't need any special cooking appliances or any special ingredients. If you do any cooking, you probably already have the things you need around your kitchen. Whatever you don't have should be readily available at your local food mart. There's nothing exotic about this.

Think back to the last time you've been to your favorite restaurant. Was there a line? When seated, how did you anxiously wait for your favorite meal to arrive? Then that feeling came when the waitress put it on the table. Finally, ahhh, was it perfect? Or was it not? Like it just wasn't cooked right. Or maybe it wasn't warm enough or they left a topping out? What did you feel when you got this bill? Did 'Aahhh' become 'woooah'? I'll show you how you can stop such problems associated with eating out. It's all by using reliable and proven copycat recipes. Want to know the top five reasons to make your favorite home-made foods?

Cost
How much do copycat recipes actually save you? Let's say you're out to eat with your significant other. Now let's add some drinks and a tip. You have invested $60-$80 comfortably anywhere in the neighborhood. You get an appetizer, two exits, and perhaps a dessert is split. You might have made the same meal at home for $25-$30, less than half the eating out price! And in the meantime, don't lose any flavor. That is a huge saving in these economic times. That sounds great but we are talking about how many recipes?

Health
That's the wonderful thing about making home copycat recipes. They give you the exact ingredients, but whatever you see fit, you can change them. Whether to give a different flavor to the food, or add your own homegrown vegetables. You can also add ingredients lower in fat, or remove ingredients to which you are allergic. The

possibilities are endless. You are in full control of that. Like the original dishes, how do you learn how these recipes taste?

Quality

A team of professional chefs created these recipes. We have checked over and over to make sure you get the exact ingredients and correct steps to make your favorite dish. You can of course go online to find recipes which claim to be copycats of popular restaurants. Yes, it's free. And it's a reason they're free. These are not real recipes for copycat purposes. They are actually not even close. I've tried a couple and to be honest, they weren't close, they weren't even good. I'll show you how to get the real copycat recipes and get your freedom back.

Freedom

Will you know how much you waste eating out of your time and freedom? Can you get the midnight meal you prefer? When watching your favorite series, will you eat your favorite meal? For instance, you are driving to the restaurant, waiting to sit down, waiting to get your appetizer, waiting to get your meal, waiting to get your dessert and, you guessed it, waiting to pay your bill. So, how much you did wait? Two hours, three more hours? Take your time and freedom back, and fix your favorite meals at home. Use these copycat recipes when you want to make your favorite meal and how you want it.

All of these dishes are custom-tested and customer-approved restaurants. Do you have an enjoyable meal at a restaurant and would like to replicate it at home? There are a few cloned restaurant recipes now, because some of you have been asking for them. Almost every one of us went to a restaurant and had a meal that was so delicious that we wanted to know how to make that meal at home. There is a staggering increase in interest in discovering online restaurants.

Have you ever wondered what the "Chef's" secrets are that made all the restaurant's famous dishes? Real Restaurant Recipes, sauce and gravy dishes, are hidden recipes for a number of sauce restaurants; each is a popular home-made dish. There's a multitude of books out there that have unnecessary copycat dishes of the popular top-secret recipes. How can I learn to cook those popular dishes in the restaurant?

Cooking also shows that there is no shortcut to performance. You can substitute less healthy ingredients for healthier ingredients when you prepare those famous restaurant recipes at home. Now, I will create my own meals and present them whenever I cook. Getting into the habit of eating at home is a hard thing, but learning how to cook your favorite restaurant meals in the comfort of your own kitchen can make it a little easier. It's not really that hard to learn how to cook secret restaurant meals. People think you need a background in cooking or a degree in culinary arts to be able to cook those secret dishes. What better way to control the consistency of what you and your family shove into your mouth than by preparing your own meals? Today, this remains the best reason to learn to cook: because you can.